NOT TODAY
Cancer

A Rockstar Chronicle of Crushing
Cancer like a BADASS

ELLEN OLSON

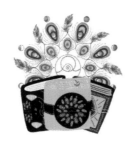

Sonoma Healing Press

With offices at
Sonoma, CA | Phoenix, AZ| | Nevada City, CA
Sonomahealingpress.com | info@sonomahealingpress.com

Print Book ISBN: 978-1-955897-15-0
Ebook ISBN: 978-1-955897-10-5

Library of Congress Cataloging-in-Publication
Data available upon request.

Book Cover Typeset Fonts
Marvel, Quartzo
KG Do You Love Me
Melancoline

Printed in the United States

A ROCKSTAR CHRONICLE OF CRUSHING CANCER LIKE A BADASS!

Contents

Dedications

I dedicate this book to Ryan Jones, my loving partner, for being my rock through one of the most terrifying experiences of my life. Thank you for doing all of the homework and research prior to all of my appointments so that I could focus on being alive. Thank you for lifting me up through my doubts and making me feel beautiful every step of the way. For always protecting me. For reading all the scary things and telling me only what I needed to hear. For all of your patience during my struggle days and for cherishing me every moment. For stepping out of your comfort zone to follow through with my shenanigans. Surviving cancer with you by my side gave our relationship strength. If we can do this together, we can pretty much do anything. I love you more than I can begin to express.

Hippy-Llove
Thank yous!!

My support team, my cartel of love, is what made this book possible. Because of the consistent support from my love cartel that included friends near and far, my group of besties, my partner, Ryan, and my family, I was able to literally skate through cancer. You all cheered me on, sent cards, gifts, prayers, Reiki healing, funded my holistic therapies, took me on walks, skated with me, had parties in my front yard, and covered my costs to live while my business was shut down during COVID. You researched information that I needed, connected me to other cancer survivors to support me, sent videos, funded my healthy meals, and so much more.

I want to thank Reggie for connecting me to the most awesome team of experts at Sutter Health and holding my hand through the most difficult parts of it.

Thank you Nancy for closing my business down. You gave me peace of mind and this allowed me to get through my treatments without stressing about packing up 13 years of equipment and memories in the midst of cancer and a pandemic.

Thank you Terrah for making sure my house was germ free and sparkling for all of my chemotherapy. Your act of kindness allowed me to relax into my space and heal without worry of getting sick.

To Claudia for hooking a sister up with delicious, organic home-cooked meals! You saved me during my worst days of chemotherapy. Thank you for the peace of mind knowing I could eat nutritious food without all the meal planning and prep work! Your food had so much love in it!

Thank you Jessa, Karina, and Absinthia for organizing the cartel of love, making sure I had rides, food and other necessities so I could rest and heal. You ladies were super pro and made it all magically happen!

To Arabella and Sassy, my inspiration and laughter through my cancer treatments. My beautiful entrepreneurs who encouraged and celebrated my pivot. You both were my muscle who would have given my cancer a beatdown if you could have!

Thank you to Nara for checking in, for coming to my aid, for initiating walks, even when I didn't want to go. I enjoyed our karaoke walks with lights and wigs and utter silliness! This lit me up on my worst days!

To everyone at Alta Bates Summit Comprehensive Cancer Center. Thank you Dr. Giuroiu for your attention to every detail. I also want to thank Elizabeth

Traugott, nurse navigator, for holding my hand the entire way through my treatments—even when you got your promotion! To Whitney, for always checking in. I always felt like I had a friend on the inside! Also, to every oncology nurse I worked with. Your compassion and attention to how you spend time with your patients made the process less frightening. I didn't feel like the dog dreading going to the vet!

To my fabulous surgeon, Dr. Kwan-Feinberg. You gave me the confidence with your enthusiasm and, truthfully, I looked forward to every visit knowing I had the space to be heard. I am still impressed by the minimal scarring and pain! Thank you for making the surgery process a whole lot less scary!

Emil at Malaya Acupuncture! Thank you for treating me to your amazing acupuncture services through my entire journey. It was because of you that I could actually function throughout my treatments! There just aren't enough words for the gratitude I have for you!

Dr. Ashyanna Sevin at Central Body Chiropractic. Thank you for your nonprofit organization, Align with Love. I was able to affordably receive services from you that were instrumental to my healing. I believe that I was able to accelerate my healing and diminish pain through your intuition and magical chiropractic services. The universe had plans for us!

To Dr. Heather Barrett, my naturopathic oncologist at Walnut Creek Naturopathic. It was an honor to work with you and Dr. Mel! Every plant medicine that you recommended gave me strength and energy through my entire journey. I even looked healthy all the way through! You helped me reach my goal of looking healthy and vibrant at the finish line, instead of looking like a deteriorating cancer patient! Your attention to bloodwork that western medicine does not offer, is imperative to my success in staying healthy beyond cancer!

And last, my parents, Marv and Connie. I can't write this without crying my eyes out. If anyone has a relationship with their parents, like I do, they understand that the need to cry on your parent's shoulder doesn't always go away. Even though you couldn't always physically be there, you were. I knew you would have taken this cancer on yourselves if you could have. It's okay, it was meant to be mine for a reason. Thank you for helping me keep my lights on and footing the bill for some of my holistic services. And for being there during surgery. It was then that I felt your pain to see your daughter going through something so scary and tragic. I was comforted by your love and presence.

And thanks to my brother Paul. We've always had a great friendship, but even more so during my cancer treatments. Thanks for listening to me and validating how much this sucked at times.

Ryan, my wonderful partner, there are not enough words or thanks for all you did, so I dedicate this book to you.

Introduction

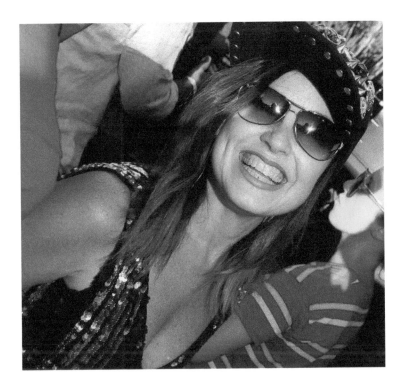

Before I was diagnosed with breast cancer, I was trying to make a career shift into wellness. I created and organized detoxes and health challenges. I assisted clients with dietary changes, but none of it fit. I love nerding out on nutrition and wellness, but found myself completely stressed about how to create a new career with all this knowledge. I didn't want to teach others how to diet. I hate the word diet! But what else was I going to do?

A voice in my head kept telling me, "You are going to go through something that will help you define your purpose in wellness."

When I was diagnosed, I realized: This is it.

Cancer is one of the number-one killers in the U.S., but does it really have to be? Can we pay attention to the reasons why it showed up? I refused to see it as a death sentence: Cancer was my life lesson.

My cancer journey was so inspiring that I wanted to share it with anyone diagnosed with a life-threatening illness. We forget that we are the boss of our bodies and we can choose whatever way we wish to heal.

I'm not here to say that my way of healing cancer is the right way. What works for me may not work for you. But I am a true testament to successfully thriving and enjoying life through my treatments. I witnessed others who had similar journeys do the same.

Just remember: You are a living, breathing human being. You still have life left in you. Be relentless and persistent. Advocate for yourself. Never back down. Take joy in learning.

This book is my personal guide to joyfully beating cancer and finishing stronger and more beautifully with a fresh new perspective than when I began.

I hope you'll find this useful in doing the same for you!

You Have a Visitor—
Its Name Is Breast Cancer

On May 18, 2020, in the middle of a pandemic that forced my business into mandatory shutdown, I got THE call that would shatter my entire world with three words, "You have cancer." As I sat on the edge of my chair while the doctor delivered this news, I began to shake and cry as the words "invasive ductile carcinoma" and "meet with a surgeon" entered my ears. OH MY GOD…INVASIVE? My heart started beating fast. I was alone. My life flashed before my eyes. The faces of two friends who had recently passed from breast cancer flashed before me. Am I going to end up dying too?

This was so unfair. After years focused on healing from too much loss, my life was really starting to come together. I had just had one of those wonderful conversations with my life partner about our future that included marriage. I didn't want to cut my time short with him! I want to grow old with this man!

The woman on the phone said, "I'm so sorry. Ellen. We are here for you." And in a moment of compassion, all I could say was, "I'm so sorry you have to deliver this kind of news. That must be so hard for you."

I couldn't believe it. I mean, aren't you supposed to feel terrible when you have cancer? Aside from the stress of closing my business down, I felt great! I started exercising more during the pandemic because I had time! I even enrolled in a course to get my group fitness certification. There's no way I could have cancer! I eat healthy, all those greens!!! I quit drinking coffee and alcohol in 2015. I am a model of wellness! My mammogram just six months prior to diagnosis was clear. How could this be?

The emotions came swirling around me like a giant tornado. I felt angry for getting cancer despite all of my healthy practices. I was so afraid of what I didn't know. I felt guilty about the emotional turmoil this would cause my friends, family, and partner. I felt guilty knowing that I would have to rely on others to help me. I knew that I would have to ask for financial help because my business was shut down and the help I received from the government was not enough to live on. I never wanted to be a burden. And now here I am, on a roller coaster that I never wanted to ride.

I was so distraught, I could barely figure out how to use my phone to call my partner, Ryan. How do I tell my life partner, the man I wanted to spend the rest of my life with that the woman he chose has breast cancer and that being with me means that over the next year we are going to endure some very stressful, scary stuff. And even then, I can't even guarantee I'm going to live. These were the dark thoughts swimming in my head at the time.

Once I was able to reach him, between crying and damn near hyperventilating, I muttered out the words, "I have cancer and it's invasive." He was silent for a moment and then said, "I'm on my way." That was the longest 30 minutes of my life.

Next on the call list was my mom. *Sigh.* This woman had just endured several years of taking care of dying loved ones. After burying her mother, dealing with her brother's suicide, and my dad's brother passing shortly after, I didn't want to deliver my cancer news to my parents. It just seemed so unfair to them.

I'm so grateful to my neighbor, who happened to be home at the time. Getting news like this while alone is horrible. She met me on the sidewalk where we embraced, and she allowed me to cry. If anyone could understand the feeling of a diagnosis, it was Nara. She had been diagnosed with breast cancer just a year before me.

My mind raced with questions: "How did this happen? Where did this come from? Is this karma? What could I have done more to prevent this? Was it all those years I drank a little too much or experimented with drugs? Did I abuse my body too much? Is this God's way of punishing me? What did I do to deserve this?!!"

When Ryan arrived, he walked straight for me, and held me tight as I hard-cried into his chest. All I could think was, "Please dear universe, don't take me away from him."

As my sobbing subsided, Ryan looked me in the eyes and said, "We're gonna beat this, Bean."

I took some deep breaths, blew my nose, wiped my tears, looked at Nara and Ryan and said, "You know what? This cancer messed with the wrong bitch."

And from that moment on, I knew that I was going to be okay.

I believed that the cancer was a messenger and that if I was going to heal, I was going to have to pay attention to what that message was. I was also going to have to be dedicated to my healing process by eating healthy, continuing to exercise, to ignite the light inside of me and turn my spirit up to 11. And although I didn't choose this disease, it chose me. And at that moment I decided to roll with it. I shook hands with my cancer and said "Okay, you are here but we're gonna do this on MY terms!"

2

Assembling the Cartel of Love

"Good friends are like stars. You don't always see them but they are always there."
—Christy Evans

After the initial shock of diagnosis comes the dreaded part of waiting for more information. Days feel like weeks, weeks feel like months. Isn't this cancer getting bigger by the second? Shouldn't something be done. Right. Now?

Lucky for me, one of my best friends, Reggie, happened to be a nurse manager for Sutter Health and had the skinny on all the best doctors and nurses available. Because of COVID, Ryan couldn't be with me during my appointments. Reggie said, "I'm gonna use my clout to get you the best team in place and meet you for your appointments so you don't have to go through this alone." This took a huge burden off of me and I KNEW she would steer me in the best direction for care. I like to think that I am strong enough to go into these appointments alone BUT I know all this information can be overwhelming. Knowing I had a friend, who understood all the medical terminology AND would take notes AND make sure I understood what was happening, was so comforting.

The next day, the nurse navigator from the breast health center where I received my biopsy called to tell me the surgeon and oncologist had been contacted and that their offices would be reaching out to me for appointments. My partner was with me at the time of the call, firing off questions to the nurse navigator. Ryan, by nature and in his profession, is a problem solver. He is the guy who helps design strategies for corporations that are in giant hot water for fraud or poor business management. He has the ability to dissect a big problem, ask the right questions, and throw a game plan onto a spreadsheet.

Thank goodness he had the ability to stay calm and put his project-managing hat on to do all the research and compose a long list of questions for my doctors' appointments because I was still in my process of accepting my cancer diagnosis! We learned that my type of cancer was called triple-negative breast cancer or TNBC for short. It is called triple-negative because it tests negative for estrogen and progesterone receptors and doesn't make too much of the protein called HER2. Well, this must be a good cancer to have, right? It doesn't test positive for hormones or HER2!" WRONG!! Triple-negative breast cancer is a crazy beast that spreads like wildfire and can metastasize quickly. But when the nurse navigator uttered the words, "This type of cancer responds very well to chemotherapy," my heart sank. Isn't chemotherapy poison? I DID NOT want to ever dump toxins into my body and suffer from lifelong side effects from chemo. I worked REALLY hard to eat a clean diet for about 10 years. I had not had a sip of alcohol in five years. I never smoked cigarettes. And now I was faced with the necessity of dumping poison in my body in order to live.

I was scheduled first to see my surgeon eight days after my diagnosis. Eight days is plenty long enough to drop into a rabbit hole of negative thoughts and Googling.

I wasn't ready to read all the nasty things about my cancer. And truthfully, I wasn't ready to deal with it. I decided that the best way I could deal with it was to clean up my diet and research the best supplements to slow down cancer growth. I continued exercising. I took the advice of my nurse navigator who told me to try to continue living my life as normal.

Live my life. Oh yes! I'm fucking alive! I better live it in the best way I know how right now!

After all, I had no idea how terrible I would feel during treatments or what kind of surgery I was having or when. There was too much uncertainty in this waiting period so I might as well make the most of it.

I was also well aware that chemotherapy was a big possibility. I had just told a friend prior to my diagnosis that one day I would likely get cancer because of my family history. Everyone on my mother's side of the family had some kind of cancer at some point. Some survived and some did not. Did saying that out loud trigger my cancer? Did the universe take this statement as a request? I decided that I'd choose my words wisely from here on out.

I began to take inventory of my life and remove anything toxic from it. How was my diet? Were there any toxic people I've been spending time with? What was I most unhappy with that I need to dispose of? It was time to let go of every single thing in my life that wasn't serving me.

I was not about to go into my cancer journey with any bullshit hanging over my head. Stress is equally as toxic as bad relationships, crappy diets, drinking too much booze, and smoking. I chose not to create an environment where cancer would be happy. This is only temporary. This cancer ain't paying rent to live inside my body and I'm not half-assing this eviction process!

Under mandatory COVID lockdown, my business of 13 years was sitting around collecting dust. I owned a cute boutique and holistic skin care salon in the thriving neighborhood of Lake Merritt in Oakland. For nearly 20 years, I spent my days in a candle-lit room, entertaining and pampering clients by giving luxurious facial and waxing treatments. For several years, I had one foot in and one foot out of my business. We had a beloved, loyal clientele, but at the same time, I grew so tired of meeting new clients and dealing with the constant boundary setting and standing my ground every time I had to enforce my policy to those who didn't show up for their appointment. No matter how you feel or what is happening in your life, in the service industry, you must pretend that those things don't exist. Headache? Take an aspirin and put on a happy face. Feeling grief? Wipe those tears, suck it up and greet that client with a smile. I grew weary of being confined to a dark room all day with ideas exploding from my mind of all things I wanted to accomplish on the outside. My passion for the industry was lost. I didn't feel challenged anymore. The amount of energy it took to work with so many different personalities and needs exhausted me. I barely could enjoy life or hang out with friends because I was completely drained of my life force.

Owning a business is hard work. The space must be maintained well. If the client has a bad experience with an employee, it was on me to fix it. If equipment malfunctioned, I had to find time between clients or stay late to repair it. Some weeks our books would be filled and I was on top of the world; other weeks were slow or filled with flaky clients who fought and refused to pay my no-show fee. Sometimes after paying all of my expenses and staff, I couldn't pay myself. It had been clear for many years that my love for my business had diminished and it was reflecting back on me as I struggled financially.

At the same time, my identity of owning this business and as a skin therapist for 20 years was coming to an end. Who was I without this identity?

Prior to my diagnosis, I had spent the last several years working with business coaches to form a new business plan and part of that plan was to sell my business. But when COVID shut all nonessential businesses down and I received my cancer diagnosis, I knew beyond a shadow of a doubt that I no longer wanted any of this hanging over my head. It was time to let go. I was ready and had been ready for years. The virus and cancer just sped up my process.

The silver lining? A large deposit from the Small Business Administration to pivot my business arrived on the date of my cancer diagnosis. I was relieved to have this money to start fresh and invest in my new business plan once I finished my cancer treatment and COVID was no longer holding us hostage. Though these were shitty circumstances all around, I gave thanks to my cancer and to COVID for creating circumstances to break me out of a box that no longer fit.

Next up, I had to assemble my army of support!

I could not allow my partner, Ryan, to take on the emotional and financial weight of my cancer journey. Because of the pandemic, he already took on the responsibility of driving me to and from my chemotherapy appointments.

I turned to friends. Over the 15 years of living in the Bay Area, I had built a solid network of amazing, loyal and loving friendships. I've witnessed the power of my community when other friends struggled through hardships. It was like being a part of a mafia, only without violence! I knew I could count on my friends and family to support me and Ryan through this not-so-great adventure.

I posted the news of my diagnosis on Facebook and was almost immediately flooded with calls and texts. My heart exploded with joy from all of the outpouring of love and support, but I couldn't keep up. Everyone wanted to help in every way. I mentioned to Ryan that it would be best to create a support group on Facebook and we could appoint a few friends to take on tasks of managing questions and areas of support. As soon as Ryan created the support page, Ellen Kicks Cancer's Ass, friends from all over the globe responded and true magic began to unfold.

A GoFundMe page was created to finance integrative therapies and my massive 7K deductible. Friends posted my GoFundMe campaign and their friends contributed. People I didn't even know sent money! I was blown away and humbled by everyone's generosity! Several weeks later, we reached our goal of 20K.

Friends requested we provide them with an Amazon wish list of necessities, which I filled with suggestions ranging from wigs, beanies, and supplements to art supplies to keep me occupied during my chemotherapy sessions. Within a matter of days of posting, packages arrived on my front porch.

My beautiful friend, Claudia, a talented vegetarian chef, volunteered to prep and cook delicious, organic meals for me. Friends in the support group began sending her money for her grocery list.

My friends contacted their friends who were cancer survivors to provide support. The women who contacted me really helped ease my fears around the treatment process. Many of these ladies spent hours chatting with me and continually checking in with me through my journey.

My sweet friend Terrah deep-cleaned my home to shining perfection before each chemo session.

Gifts showed up on my doorstep. Cards arrived in the mail. Friends who threw online events posted my GoFundMe page to get more donations. The outpouring of love rushed in and never once stopped. My support page consisted of cancer survivors, nurses, doctors, social workers, project managers, attorneys, artists, holistic practitioners, and so many more. If and when I needed assistance, we had it covered.

This outpouring of love and assistance was humbling and overwhelmingly beautiful. Even just a quarter of what I received was beyond expectations. I felt like I was the untouchable mob boss and every person in my love cartel was going to bat for me and I didn't even have to lift a finger.

Ryan spent time researching everything about my cancer as I was just not ready to see all the scary statistics.

The biggest task was closing down my two-story business of 13 years. And while I was so ready to say goodbye, the idea of packing up 13 years of memories and my entire identity felt too unbearable to handle while in the midst of appointments, emotional break-downs, and chemotherapy. Another one of my besties, Nancy, came to the rescue. She sold off all of my assets for more than I would have even asked, enlisted help in organizing boxes, packed up the tiny amount of items left over, moved it all out into storage, and met with the landlord for a final walk-through and key exchange. Within a month after moving the rest of the items to storage, she sold everything else off and we were able to cancel the storage unit and remove that expense. This incredible act of kindness reduced my stress 100%.

While everyone was busy making my life easier, I put my nutrition education to work, researching all the possible healing remedy options. I researched naturopathic oncologists to help support my body through chemotherapy and surgery.

My amazing acupuncturist, who I had been working with for nearly four years, offered free services to me throughout my cancer treatments.

I ordered a PEMF (pulsed electromagnetic field) mat that also combined infrared heat and photon therapy to accelerate healing, detoxify, and soothe aches and pains. I will explain the benefits of this magical healing mat later in this book.

I needed inspiration and books to keep me from living in fear. Where were the success stories and holistic healers? I purchased Jane McClelland's *How to Starve Cancer* and *The Metabolic Approach to Cancer* by Dr. Nasha Winters and Jess Higgins Kelley. These books focused on dietary guidelines to help heal cancer.

A friend of mine also gifted me the book *Radical Remission: Surviving Cancer Against All Odds* By Kelly A. Turner. This is a beautiful book filled with real stories from cancer survivors who were literally delivered a death sentence by their western doctors and took an integrative approach to healing, eliminating their cancer for good. Those who were interviewed had outlived their cancer diagnosis 10 years and beyond. I also bought the audiobook so that I could listen when I was driving or doing tasks. This book helped me breathe. It empowered and uplifted me. It gave me strength and helped me believe that I could live well beyond the life expectancy of a stage 4, triple-negative breast cancer diagnosis.

Next Up—Spiritual Guidance

I grew up in the Catholic Church. Our family dressed up and attended church every Sunday. To say that my elder and younger brother tolerated church would be an understatement. It was hard enough to not poke fun at each other and to maintain good behavior! In our later teen years, I remember having a family powwow and my father announcing, "I know you kids aren't really happy about going to church and that's okay. What I hope for you is that you find your own spiritual practice. You can become a Buddhist, Mormon, or join a Baptist church as long as you can pray."

Truthfully, I feared God. What I learned from my years sitting in a pew, is that if you fuck up, you were going to hell: No heavenly sandbox for you. But if you were good, you got to go to heaven. Uh, God, aren't you the perfect one? Doesn't it say somewhere in the bible that you're perfect and we are imperfect? By definition, we were bound to fuck up.

Around the time of my second divorce, I spent a lot of time working on myself through therapy and reading every single book on personal growth I could get my hands on. I started reading *The Artist's Way*. What I didn't know was that this book would help me find my spiritual path.

3

Overcoming the Brain Weasels

"Fear does not stop death. It stops life."

—Vi Keeland

ancer diagnosis can really fuck with your brain. I questioned every single method of care I used to save my life. Am I doing enough? Or am I doing too much? Am I wasting my money? Or do I need to spend more on this other treatment? What if I eat a little sugar? Is this bag of grapes going to make my cancer come back? I don't want to eat this salad; I want to eat pizza and ice cream. But will I literally be committing suicide by indulging a little bit? WHAT IF ALL THIS DOESN'T WORK?

I worry about dying ahead of Ryan and what that would do to him. I didn't want to hurt him. I didn't want him to find someone else and forget me. I didn't want to be replaced. I would miss kisses, nose nuzzles, and holding hands when we sleep. I would miss dancing under the sun with him and making our plans for world domination. I would miss all of his jokes about my being tiny and me teasing him about being grumpy. I would miss stealing bites of his food and terrifying each other with our farts. I would miss the honest communication we have. I would miss having new experiences with him. I would miss being with someone who makes me feel so important, treats me like a queen, protects and cherishes me. I would miss his late-night soapbox rants. He is a true gem, a rare find, my person who balances my energy and insanity, my rock. He is beautiful inside and out and while we are truly opposite, we are a match made in heaven.

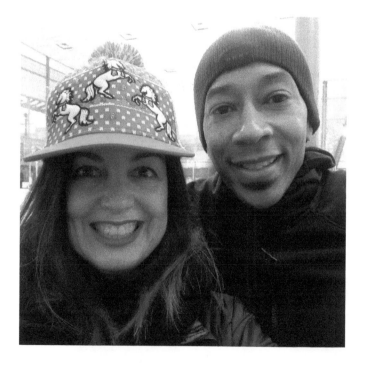

We had just started making our life plans together, and wham, my cancer diagnosis!

I felt sad for my parents who might have to endure the fear and grief of losing their child. I wished I had never moved away. I wished I had more time with them. I thought about all the traveling I could have done or how I spent more time in a job I didn't want to be in. And of course, maybe I wouldn't have cancer if I hadn't put myself through that stress.

Why did I stay in a job that took so much energy that I couldn't even enjoy time with friends? I felt like I fucked up so badly at life. My life didn't go as planned. I wanted to travel and go on more camping trips. Why didn't I give myself more time off?

Fuck. I totally gave myself this cancer. This is my fault.

I had to train myself to speak to my internal chatter. I would simply say, "Thank you for your input, subconscious. Yes, we have lessons to learn from this cancer, but you did not deliberately try to kill yourself. We are alive and well today and will keep putting 100% effort into healing. All you can do is your very best." I found it very important to talk to my internal chatter. It is possible to change your thought patterns, and doing so is an act of self love. Acknowledging fear and embracing yourself can be healing. Letting yourself know that you have your back is empowering. Think of it like a higher power telling you that they understand your fear, but that you are held, you are not alone, and you have the power to overcome this scary thing. That feels good, doesn't it?

4

Assembling the Western Medicine Cartel

Tossing the grenade at cancer.

The Surgery Strategy

Eight days after my initial diagnosis, I met with my surgeon. Reggie came along with me and had made a cute three-ring binder that says, "Ellen Kicks Cancer's Ass" with a photo of me jumping in the air.

The notebook was to be brought to all of my appointments for note-taking, adding in all of my visit summaries and handouts.

The medical staff at Carol Ann Read Breast Health Center had highly recommended my surgeon. Whenever I mentioned her name to anyone who knew her, everyone sang her praises. Reggie also informed me that she would work hard to get her on my team.

Because of the pandemic, Ryan was not allowed to attend my appointment, but we were able to set up a conference call with him. I showed up in good spirits with my laptop, ready to tackle this cancer. Reggie and I were called into the examination room, and after the nurse asked a few questions and checked my vitals and weight, she had me disrobe and wait for the doctor.

We set up my laptop and dialed up Ryan and then began cracking jokes and laughing. I'm sure you could hear us throughout the entire floor. We heard a knock on the door, and I stood up and said, "Oh shit, we are being too noisy." My surgeon walked in all smiles and was friendly. She said, "You're okay, laughter is good!"

Instead of going right into the specifics, she said, "I want to learn about you. Tell me what kinds of things you like to do and what your lifestyle is like. What do you do for work?"

I explained to her about closing down my holistic skin care salon of 13 years due to COVID. I spoke of my healthy lifestyle, that I didn't smoke or drink. I expressed my love for dancing, roller skating, and being active. We talked a little about how Reggie and I became friends and how Ryan and I met. It felt more like I was hanging out with a new friend who was getting to know more about me, and that felt comforting.

She wanted to make sure that she could collect as much information about me personally, so that she knew what kind of a patient she was dealing with and to also recommend services that might be beneficial during my cancer journey.

She fully supported my holistic health practice and encouraged it. And then she said, "The cancer center provides nutrition services, provides free yoga classes and massage, and they also have an acupuncturist on board. Let's work on getting you booked for all of it!" This was music to my ears. Both Reggie and Ryan clapped and cheered with both enthusiasm and relief!. They understood how important the lifestyle support was to me. I had read horror stories about oncologists and surgeons firing their patients because their egos couldn't handle someone who knew more about nutrition and alternative therapies than they did.

My surgeon went on to explain the process. Since the cancer had clearly spread to my lymph nodes, I would have to start with chemotherapy to shrink the cancer before surgery could be done.

She said, "I have good news. Triple-negative cancer responds very well to chemotherapy and usually wipes the cancer out."

I began to cry. Chemotherapy, the one thing I didn't want to do, was the one thing that could save my life. But because she was so encouraging, I was sold.

My surgeon then performed an ultrasound to get a good idea of what we were dealing with and to record the size of the tumors.

"We will need you to get a breast MRI and a PET scan. The PET scan will let us know whether the cancer has spread to any other organs. You will be meeting with your oncologist to go over all of your chemotherapy treatment and, at some point during your chemotherapy, you will meet with a radiation oncologist about your radiation treatments. At this time, we can't stage your cancer until we know what the PET scan tells us."

Oof. Radiation. I really don't know if I want to do that. Can I skip it? I guess I'll see what my oncologist has to say.

"We will need to schedule you for surgery to place a port under your skin on your right side. The port allows access for blood draws and to administer your chemo and other medications. We do this so we aren't sticking you with needles all the time. Also, because you will be sitting during chemotherapy for several hours, this allows your hands and arms to be free. It can be placed on the inner side of your right breast kind of in your cleavage area or around near where your bra strap would be just above your right breast.

While my surgeon was very encouraging, there was still so much we didn't know. But I did feel like I was in good hands with her and that she would have my back throughout this journey.

Two days later, I had my breast MRI done and the day after that, my PET scan. Within 24 hours of getting the PET scan, my surgeon called with the results, and I am so thankful that Ryan was with me to share the news.

"Ellen, the good news on your breast MRI is that the cancer has not spread to your right breast. You do have some type of a cyst there but doesn't appear to be cancer. I can biopsy this cyst when I surgically implant your port. Your PET scan shows a lot of cancer activity in your left breast. There are lymph nodes in your chest wall that are showing cancer and four lymph nodes under your arm. Your breast tumor is about 3.5 cm (about 1.38 inches) and your top sentinel lymph node is 2.8 cm (about 1.10 inches). The second lymph node is 1.4 cm (a little over half an inch) and there appears to be cancer in your trachea that measures 1 cm (about the size of a pea). There is a tumor on your liver, but we don't know what that is. It's not lighting up as cancer."

I began to shake. "What stage do you think I am?"

"Well, if this cancer is really in your trachea, then this would put you at stage 4."

Tears rolled down my face. "Okay."

I know Ryan asked her some questions, but I don't even know what he said. Everything switched to mute.

I fell to the floor and began to sob.

"How did this happen? How did it get so bad? How did it get into my trachea!! What the fuck is on my liver?!!"

As I lay in a puddle on the floor, Ryan held me and then at one point stood up, grabbed my boxing gloves and handed them to me. He placed the boxing pads on his hands and said, "C'mon, Bean. Start punching and yell. Get mad. C'mon, get up and punch it out."

It was a sunny day. My windows were open.

I began punching those pads as hard as I could yelling every curse word in the book. I punched and screamed obscenities until I couldn't punch anymore. And then I dropped to the floor and cried. "What am I gonna do?"

"We're gonna fight like hell," he said.

Oncology—A Lesson in Chemical Warfare

Fourteen days after my initial diagnosis, I met with my oncologist on June 1st. Ryan was allowed to come for my first visit. I was so glad because he was always 10 steps ahead, always knowing what questions to ask. I was still hanging on for dear life, trying to keep myself from sliding off a steep cliff.

Reggie also joined in so that she could introduce me to some of her old coworkers who would also help me along my journey. With Reggie at my side, my mind was more at ease. If Ryan and I couldn't understand something, she would break it down for us.

As we waited in the very somber waiting room, I noticed the other waiting patients. Some wore caps, others just looked exhausted. I hoped that during my cancer journey I didn't look anywhere near how they must have felt. You could see that their treatment had beat them down and that the energy it took to get to their appointment took everything that they had left. Was this my destiny?

I was first greeted by my nurse navigator, Elizabeth. At my cancer center, nurse navigators are the support, voice of reason, and the person you report to for any issues related to your treatments during your cancer journey. Even if you had questions about anything out of her zone, she would find the right person to assist you. To me, it was everything to know that I had someone at the cancer center who could be my rock.

I felt like this was my first day of school. Elizabeth led Ryan, Reggie and me to a conference room and set up several chairs in a circle. Was I going to have to stand up and say, "Hello, my name is Ellen and I have breast cancer." I felt like I was attending an intervention! Turns out, in addition to me, Reggie, Ryan, Elizabeth, and my oncologist, a few others would be joining us. It was kind of like a gang initiation, but for cancer.

Next, Reggie's friend Whitney, the cancer center's nurse practitioner, entered the room. We both realized that we had met previously at an event in Oakland with Reggie. I began to feel like I had a team of good girlfriends on my side! The nurse manager, Laura, also Reggie's friend and old co-worker, came to introduce herself and assured me if I ever needed anything she was there to help.

Once we were all seated, my oncologist arrived. She was young, petite with dark hair, and had an accent that I couldn't place. Later I found out she is Romanian. She didn't waste any time and got right down to business. Her style was much different from my surgeon's. My surgeon was fun and cheerful with a winning attitude. My oncologist had a giant list of detailed events to go over and there was no time to waste.

I was nervous. Was she going to tell me I had six months to live? Or that these treatments would buy me a few years? I couldn't bear to hear it, so I kind of tuned out.

All I really got out of our meeting was that I would have to endure five solid months of chemotherapy. My healthy tissues would be destroyed. All of the work for my health was about to be destroyed. Every strand of my hair on my body would fall out. My skin would get dry, my nails might turn purple or black and fall off. My white counts would drop. I might have severe nausea, diarrhea, or vomiting. But I would get anti-nausea meds to remedy the sickness that would cause severe constipation. I could end up having bone pain. I would be thrown into menopause. Oh joy! No more periods! One fucking silver lining! As she listed off the side effects, I held back the tears. Why the fuck do I have to go through this?

It took about 30 minutes for her to finish going through my treatment plan. "Do you have any questions?" I was numb. This woman is telling me that by the time I finish chemo, I'll become an old, hairless, lifeless prune with menopausal hot flashes, mood swings, and brittle bones.

Now my goals of entering into 50 with six-pack abs are ruined. Goodbye beach body. Hello hairless waif.

I looked to my right at Ryan, knowing he would have questions to fire off at her. He was checking things off of his list. I'm so glad that he's able to keep it together enough to research everything and understand what questions to ask. And thank goodness that he's the type of guy who sees me for more than the way I look.

What we did find out that day is that my oncologist had plans to take my PET scans to have a group of doctors review it. Turns out she's not sure if the cancer has spread to my trachea.

At the end of our meeting, Elizabeth said, "I know this is a lot to take in, but I'm going to set aside some time for us to go over your treatment plan in detail along with side effects. We'll also get you a calendar set up for your chemotherapy and medicine schedule." Thank goodness. Because it was a lot to take in. I'm still in denial. There's a chance that this might be a horrible dream, right?

The best part about this entire meeting was that my oncologist did not give me a life expectancy. She didn't tell me I was going to die. She didn't discuss statistics and mortality rates. What she did tell me was that she had developed a plan to reduce my cancer and maybe even demolish it completely. And that she and her staff would be with me all the way. I could now walk out of this meeting with more certainty that I could beat this.

A few days later, I met with Elizabeth. She gave me handouts that I could refer to about each chemotherapy drug I would be receiving. She also gave me a calendar of my chemo infusion dates along with a schedule of when I had to take my prescription drugs that were to give me relief from the side effects of chemo. Elizabeth informed me that the anti-nausea medications are so good that the majority of patients don't have to deal with vomiting or nausea. I was so happy to hear this. While I accepted that vomiting and nausea were a part of the package, I wasn't thrilled that I'd have to endure that part of the side effects. Fingers crossed that I'd be one of the lucky ones who wouldn't have to suffer. Many other survivors who had offered to speak to me told me the same: They never vomited and only experienced mild nausea. If I stayed on top of taking my anti-nausea meds, I wouldn't have to be crying with my head in the toilet for days on end!

Elizabeth also informed me that I would be highly toxic for up to three days after my infusion. This meant that I had to keep my used bath towels away from Ryan. Anyone who did my laundry had to wear gloves.

We were also told that slobbery make-out sessions could contaminate Ryan and possibly make him sick. And should we have the urge to have sex, we had to wear condoms. WHO THE FUCK GETS HORNY DURING CHEMOTHERAPY? I mean, how does anyone feel sexy going through all of these side effects? But I guess it happens. And that's why before every infusion, I had to do a pregnancy test. My hat is off to anyone getting laid during chemo!

First Surgery—The Port Catheter, the Device That Delivers the Chemotherapy

I was not excited about having a device inserted beneath my skin. How was I going to exercise? I'm a wild sleeper! Am I going to wake up in pain from being in a weird sleeping position? I guess I won't know if I and this port are going to get along until I recover from surgery.

Reggie just so happened to work in the exact hospital where I was having my port surgery. Again, because of the pandemic, Ryan couldn't assist me or even come inside. He nervously drove me to the hospital, parked and walked me to the entrance where Reggie was waiting for me. I could sense his worries and I knew it was tearing him up inside. It was abundantly clear that he detested the idea of me being in pain. If he could have stood over the surgeon, asking questions the entire time and directing her to do it right, he would have. If anyone made any mistakes throughout this process, he would find out where this person lived and burn their house down. It was like having my own mafia boss on my side. No one had better fuck up or fuck with this man's Bean. This man is more than my love, he is my best friend, my protection, my knight, my person who cherishes and respects me. And dammit, nothing and no one would ever hurt me. Not on his watch.

Reggie assured Ryan that I was in great hands and that my surgeon was THE best. Before going inside, I hugged my goodbyes and told him everything would be okay. That hug felt like no other. I know in his mind he was praying hard.

The entire process for this surgery wouldn't take more than an hour. I wasn't going under anesthesia, but just a gentle twilight anesthetic, which means I wouldn't be knocked out, just gently sedated.

As Reggie and I walked towards the surgery check-in, everyone greeted her. She knew damn near everyone that passed us as well as the folks working in surgery registration. Once I arrived, I was checked in, weighed, and vitals taken. Once I passed those tests, I was given a gown to change into. Reggie wasn't allowed to hang out with me prior to surgery so we said our goodbyes and she promised to check in when I was in recovery. I was taken back to the pre-surgery area and given a nice, warm bed and covered in toasty blankets.

I was greeted by a couple of nurses who checked me in and administered my IVs.

About an hour after I was checked in, my surgeon came to visit me, all smiles and cheerful. She pulled up my PET scan and said, "Ellen, I have great news! You've been downgraded to a stage 3C. The board discussed your case and said that this trachea area wasn't lighting up like all the other areas that have cancer. We believe that the area that is lighting up is a lymph node that is very close to your trachea."

Stage 3C??? This sounds way better than a stage 4 diagnosis!!!! This was the first time that I had ever seen what a PET scan looked like. And seeing all those cancer spots in my breast and lymph nodes still left me feeling uneasy.

My surgeon took notice of the look on my face and said with total confidence, "Ellen, I just know you are gonna beat this."

My eyes welled up with tears, "I feel it too." I said.

And with that she got up and said, "I'll see you in surgery!"

My anesthesiologist showed up just a few minutes after and explained that I would be lightly sedated and wouldn't feel anything. I would wake up feeling well rested. Awesome! I could use some restful moments! I think he must have given me something prior to wheeling me to surgery because by the time we got to the operating room, I pretty much passed out.

I awoke to hearing the voice of my surgeon and sounds of scissors snipping something. I gently opened my eyes and it appeared she was bandaging me up. "You did great, Ellen! We're all finished! We're gonna wheel you to recovery!"

I spent about 90 minutes in recovery and going over my post-care directions with one of the nurses in recovery. And the best part? They let Reggie come back to see me! The only issue was that my surgeon contacted Ryan to let him know I was finished so he had been waiting in the parking lot for over an hour thinking something awful had happened. When really, I was just in the midst of all the post-op procedures. Unfortunately, my phone was locked up somewhere and I had no way to contact him.

Once they decided to release me, Reggie was allowed to wheel me in a wheelchair out to where Ryan was waiting to pick me up. At that point I was completely alert and ready to go home and relax.Ryan, who was always prepared for the worst-case scenario, was surprised that I was alert, chatty and in good spirits. Poor guy was so worried something went wrong after surgery, so I'm sure it put him at ease to see that I was such a chatterbox.

Now, I was ready for chemo.

It took a while to get used to my port and, in the beginning, I wasn't allowed to lift anything heavy and was limited for the first four to six weeks in certain yoga movements and couldn't do any upper-body work-outs. But I still went on hikes and would jump on my reformer or modify my movements in yoga until my body became acclimated. After that, I could do most anything.

I understood the need for this port, but I never really became friends with it. After some time, it became less noticeable to me and didn't get in the way of much except for when I had to use a seatbelt. Occasionally, I would wear a tank top and Ryan would notice it and he would say, "Oh my poor Bean." It was a reminder for him of what I had to go through: This device was implanted so I could have toxins dumped into my body to kill off a beastly cancer.

5

Setting Boundaries

*"Daring to set boundaries is about having
the courage to love ourselves even when
we risk disappointing others"—Brene Brown*

Once the cat was out of the bag, friends came out from everywhere, even from behind bushes to offer love and support. The love came from far and wide! I knew that every single person in my cartel of love would go to bat for me no matter what. At the same time, all that love can be very overwhelming.

Texts came in day and night. There were a lot of people putting me in touch with other breast cancer survivors. People wanted to connect me with doctors and other health practitioners, cannabis experts, and others who have the knowledge to help a cancer patient. The information comes at the speed of light and sifting through it feels like full-time research. I didn't want to focus on cancer every moment of the day. I also had living to do.

All the unsolicited advice was frustrating. People want to be useful because otherwise they are helpless. I was their friend, and I was in pain so even if they had no clue, they tried to help. Sorry, but dabbing lavender and taking a teaspoon of local honey is not a cure for temporary treatment, side effects, or even cancer. But people feel better if they can help. I learned very quickly that I had to understand my own needs first, ask for what I needed specifically, and set hard boundaries.

At times I would feel guilty. I didn't want anyone to feel bad for offering help. But sometimes the best thing that can be done in lieu of advice is to listen and validate how much something sucks. I loved random texts or videos that I would receive of someone's dogs doing something insane. Kind words and gestures filled me and did in fact make me feel better.

The Facebook support page was my saving grace since I could direct all questions and love posts directly to the page and look at them when I had the time, rather than be bombed with calls and texts. I wanted to make sure all my health practitioners' calls didn't get lost amongst all of the texts and that my team leaders could easily get in touch with me as they made arrangements to help out.

Since people from far away couldn't help in person, I made lists of things I would need throughout my cancer treatments. On that list were supplements, wigs, caps and scarves, and beauty supplies like false eyelashes and brow fillers. If I ran out of things, I would continue to add more to the list and post to my support page.

I enlisted about five people who were each in charge of one particular event to organize. That way, if anyone wanted to help, they would chat with the person organizing. For instance, one person would be in charge of organizing friends who would run errands for me during the week. Another friend would organize ride dates and times when Ryan needed a break. If I needed someone to research something for me, I would make a list of items to Google so that I wouldn't have to encounter again the long list of crappy statistics about triple-negative breast cancer.

I had to ask people to stop sending gifts that I didn't ask for because my cottage was too small to house a bunch of things that couldn't be used for healing purposes. If I made an announcement about not feeling well, I had to specifically ask everyone not to give unsolicited health advice. Anyone who didn't respect my wishes was usually met with messages from other friends from the support group to be respectful of my wishes.

It is NOT okay for anyone to give medical advice who doesn't understand the cancer journey, the medicines and supplementation involved. THIS was probably my biggest frustration, but I had to understand, too, that friends felt completely helpless and wanted nothing more than to take my discomfort away.

I also had to be clear that I would not always answer texts. While I really enjoyed all the loving messages, I just couldn't spend all day responding. I had to also set boundaries for myself to not respond and to remind myself that people weren't expecting it and wouldn't be hurt if I didn't. Setting boundaries doesn't mean we don't appreciate the help that others have to offer, we just want to keep the experience as simple and easy as possible. The people who respect that are your true friends. Anyone who doesn't understand does not deserve an explanation. No one has time for another person's selfishness or drama when you are fighting cancer. It is also not your job to babysit anyone else's emotions around your journey.

6

Assembling My Integrative Cartel

"Nature itself is the best physician."—Hippocrates

I was NOT going to go into this journey without supporting my body in all the ways I could in order to stand strong at the end of my treatments. I have no patience for feeling crappy and if I could control the outcome, well, then I would sign up for everything that resonated with me.

About 11 years prior to my diagnosis, I decided to work with a naturopath after my western doc misdiagnosed me with depression. At the time, I was having abnormally heavy periods, insomnia, eczema, and weight gain. I assumed it was a hormonal imbalance. That western doctor literally spent 10 minutes with me to come to the conclusion that I was suffering from depression. That diagnosis didn't sit right with me. I had energy; I wasn't questioning life. I didn't struggle to get out of bed every day. I was having a combination of symptoms that, no doubt in my mind, was hormonal.

I wanted a second opinion from someone who could examine my diet, lifestyle, family history and so on. I explored the internet, searching for a naturopath who specializes in women's health. Berkeley Naturopathic came highly recommended through Google and Yelp and, after booking my appointment, I understood why! The questionnaire that I filled out prior to my appointment took me about an hour to complete. The appointment took two hours as my naturopath reviewed and made detailed notes of my diet and lifestyle. She concluded that I had adrenal fatigue. She placed me on an anti-inflammatory diet, gave me a few supplements, and told me to stop training for marathons. Within just one month, my periods started returning to normal, I dropped eight pounds, began sleeping like a baby, and my eczema went away. The power of supplementation and diet are THAT powerful.

After my cancer diagnosis, I contacted my naturopath who referred me to someone who specialized in oncology. In the meantime, I was doing tons of homework on mistletoe therapy and high-dose Vitamin C IV infusions. As soon as I was diagnosed with cancer, I completely removed sugar, saturated fats, dairy, gluten, and processed foods. Truthfully, during the pandemic, I had put on an extra seven or eight pounds, just from all the take-out I ordered.

I switched to salads, using lemon and olive oil and steamed veggies, topping them off with organic vegan butter made with cashews. I also juiced at least once a day. The weight began falling off and my energy went through the roof. What aches and pains I had disappeared. Again, plants possess magical healing powers and although I missed eating chilled Reese's Peanut Butter Cups, I would prefer the long-term positive impact of this new diet.

I switched to filtered water and even put a filter on my shower to remove chemicals.I bought a pulsed electromagnetic field mat to lie on daily so that I could increase detoxification, relieve pain, and accelerate cellular healing.

I had benefited from acupuncture in the past and had a wonderful acupuncturist, Emil, who was like family to me. I had been receiving treatment from him off and on for four years but had fallen off the wagon. I suppose I had let life get in the way and had stopped doing a lot of my health-support therapies. My friend Jessa found Emil years ago and was blown away by how much better she felt after his treatments. In the end, through his herbal concoctions and acupuncture treatments, he had resolved most of her health issues.

So I began seeing Emil for my terrible digestive distress and insomnia. At that time, I was dealing with a lot of grief and anxiety. Because of Emil's treatments I began sleeping better and my digestion improved as long as I stayed on top of my healthy eating plan. My mental state had really improved and I would leave his office feeling on top of the world.

Jessa and I told everyone we could about Emil. In fact, I talked about Emil so much that a friend thought that Emil must be the name of my boyfriend. Jessa and I got a big kick out of it. When Jessa and I would get together, our partners would laugh when we brought up Emil. It was like he was the only other acceptable man in our lives.

When I got my cancer diagnosis, Jessa had prepared Emil, letting him know I'd be contacting him.I made my appointment online and showed up in his office. "I know Jessa warned you that I have cancer." I went on to explain the type of cancer I had and the current (western) treatments. "I'm hoping acupuncture can support me and help ease nausea, appetite loss, and fatigue."

As he listened, he could not mask his concern. But I knew he possessed the magic tools to get me through. "Don't you worry, Ellen. I've got you. Let's get you coming in weekly during your treatments. And don't you worry, I will treat you for free until you get on your feet."

"Oh Emil, that's so sweet! My friends raised money to help."

"Use your money for your other medical bills. You've sent me so much business in the past, that I'm happy to do this for you as a thank-you."

My heart almost exploded. I was so eternally grateful for his generosity. It gave me so much peace through my cancer journey. I always brought my meditation music and would relax, do deep breathing and meditation on his table.

Each week, he would check my pulse and listen for various weaknesses. Many times, he would treat me for appetite loss. I came to one appointment nauseated and unable to eat. Upon finishing treatment, I walked out of his building and could smell the taco trucks. I instantly wanted to eat a giant plate of tacos. In addition, I had the energy to cook. So, I made my own, healthy taqueria version and scarfed down two delicious organic vegan tacos!

We focused on insomnia, fatigue, purifying blood, lowering inflammation, detoxification, and digestive distress. I believe Emil's services truly helped me to recover from chemotherapy quickly and allowed me to stay comfortable through all of my treatments.

My previous naturopath directed me to an amazing naturopathic oncologist. She was fluent in all of the western standard-of-care treatments for cancer and understood the holistic medicine that would complement my treatments.

While I was well versed in nutrition, knowing what foods would best support me, I knew that there would be contraindications to certain supplements that might interfere with my treatment. I did not want to make any mistakes.

Reggie sat next to me during my first video meeting with my naturopath. My diet consisted of all the cancer fighting foods. I was eating tons of organic cruciferous vegetables, about three servings of fruit daily. I had also eliminated refined sugars and processed foods. With Claudia delivering healthy meals, I was set!!

My naturopathic oncologist also ordered blood tests to get a better understanding of what vitamins and minerals I might be deficient in that are directly linked to breast cancer as well as inflammatory markers. If my inflammation was up, then we had to work hard on getting that down. For me, I knew that I needed to focus on stress reduction.

When the blood tests came back, we met online again to discuss the results. My iodine levels were terribly low, my ferritin levels were extremely high, and my inflammatory markers were way up. I was also low in selenium. Looking at these blood tests alone, without even knowing I had cancer, would have indicated some type of disease. The goal was to get those inflammatory markers down, strengthen my immune system, and get my iodine numbers to go up. I wasn't sure how anyone could do this during chemotherapy, but I was willing to do whatever it took. The supplements that she prescribed would support me through chemotherapy, help to reduce inflammation, and get my iodine numbers to go up.

Of course, I always discussed my holistic therapies with my oncologist. One thing I loved about working with her and her team is that they respected my wish to integrate holistic therapies into my nine months of western treatments. I would bring evidence-based information to back up why I was using them; her team would make sure the supplementation wouldn't interfere with treatment, and generally be given thumbs up. Much of my antioxidant and DNA-building supplements had to be removed during radiation. But other than that, I was never questioned about it. I've heard so many nightmare stories from other breast cancer survivors who were actually fired by their oncologists because they wanted to integrate holistic therapies. I was so grateful that I never had that problem.

My Complete Supplement Regimen

Modified Citrus Pectin—Helps prevent the spread of cancer, lowers inflammation, and aids in removal of toxic heavy metals.

Curcumin—Curcumin is the active ingredient in turmeric and has powerful anti-inflammatory and antioxidant effects. This ingredient is what gives turmeric its reputation for being so good. However, turmeric on its own is not that powerful, so a good curcumin supplement can truly help with reducing swelling and pain. In addition, it provides cellular protection!

I-throid Iodine supplement—While my thyroid revealed no issues, having low iodine can cause thyroid disease down the road. Low iodine also increases the risk of breast cancer and, going forward, I wanted to avoid recurrence.

Astragalus—Helps to improve immune function, boost energy, and raise white blood counts. White blood counts are responsible for fighting off infection and other illnesses. This was crucial because throughout my cancer treatments my white counts would drop pretty drastically. And it was especially important for increasing my counts once I was finished with chemotherapy.

Annato E—A Vitamin E supplement that uses a unique blend of Vitamin E that isn't readily available in food. It helps to decrease inflammation, has anti-cancer benefits, prevents oxidation of cells, and promotes good skin health. This particular supplement was used more to assist with cell protection during chemotherapy and to reduce the oxidizing effects of radiation exposure.

Chaga, Turkey Tail, and Reishi mushrooms—I could spend a lot of time discussing the benefits of mushrooms. They are powerful antioxidants and contain a high content of beta-glucan which has been known to reduce tumor activity and is an exceptional weapon for strengthening immune function. Mushrooms are also amazing for digestive health and fighting off infections. They also aid in decreasing the horrible side effects of chemotherapy and help with wound healing from radiation. I did not take all of these mushrooms in a blend. I would alternate supplementation of each type of mushroom. For instance, I would take turkey tail mushrooms for a month or two and then switch to reishi and then to chaga. I would also use them in my cooking as well. Lion's mane is one of my most favorite to eat as it truly soaks up the flavors of seasonings used in cooking.

Zinc sulfate—Strengthens immune function and supports wound healing. It has been beneficial for eye function, especially useful during chemotherapy as chemo does deteriorate eyesight. Thankfully, because of all of the supplement support, my eyes were only temporarily affected.

Melatonin—There are so many studies on the use of high-dose melatonin to assist in the reduction of tumor growth. I struggle with sleep as many other perimenopausal, and menopausal women do. This can be detrimental to health over time. Melatonin can help reset your circadian rhythms that regulate healthy sleep patterns. I found that taking high-dose melatonin for several months gave me very restless sleep and night-mares. At smaller doses, 3 mg, my sleep improved. High-dose melatonin (20 mg and over) is not for everyone but can be extremely beneficial in fighting cancer.

B-12—Adenosylcobalamin/Methylcobalimin protects nerves and aids in cellular energy production. This was perfect support during chemotherapy to prevent nerve damage and/or neuropathy and was supportive during radiation against nerve pain as well.

B-3/Niacinamide—Useful for supporting the skin against inflammation and dehydration. I used this during radiation to fight against burning and oxidative stress.

B-6—Helps to treat anemia and raise hemoglobin, a consistent issue during cancer treatments. There have been studies associated with lowering risks of certain types of cancers.

Pure Honokiol—Helps with cognitive function, improving mood, reducing anxiety, and promoting relaxation. I used this for sleep and brain fog associated with chemotherapy.

Liposomal Vitamin D3/K1/K2—While my levels tested as normal at the time I started chemotherapy, they did fall during the winter. I also believe because I wasn't able to go outside due to the air quality from wildfires, this also caused my Vitamin D to drop. Vitamin D is essential for immune function, healthy bones and, when low, can put you at high risk for cancer.

Om Energy Powder—This drink helped to regulate my energy and also helped reduce brain fog. It is loaded with beta-glucan from their mushroom blend and also B vitamins to sustain energy. Guarana also helps to reduce the fatigue related to chemotherapy. The powder contains caffeine. I used only one scoop, which had about 45 mg of caffeine total. Because it has Vitamin C in it, it is not advised to use during radiation.

Mistletoe injections—Yes! This is the plant that you kiss under during the holidays! But it has amazing immune-boosting benefits and can reduce the side effects of cancer treatments. Because cancer treatments damage DNA, there are studies that have shown that mistletoe can repair damaged DNA. Mistletoe can destroy. The best way to receive mistletoe is intravenously or through injections. I did my own subcutaneous injections in my abdomen. Its use is definitely not for the faint-hearted. I spent about one third of my life getting allergy injections so dealing with needles was not a problem. My naturopathic oncologist ordered my mistletoe and provided a class on how to do injections. It was absolutely easy. The goal is to have a skin reaction, which indicates that your immune system is firing up.

Vitamin C infusions—High-dose Vitamin C infusions for me were extremely supportive during chemotherapy. When used together with chemotherapy, the Vitamin C at high dose causes oxidative stress to the cell, creating hydrogen peroxide, making a horrible environment for cancer to survive. I would get my infusions the day after chemotherapy and, typically, I would feel tired the next day and then get a boost of energy by the time Friday rolled around. I believe it also helped me with sleep. There is a lot of controversy around whether or not it is complementary to chemotherapy because oncologists have learned that Vitamin C is an antioxidant that provides cell protection. In their minds, Vitamin C won't work with chemotherapy because it would protect against the oxidative stress of chemotherapy. But what they don't understand is that higher intravenous doses cause further oxidative stress, making it a great combination with chemo. What I do know for sure is that it helped improve my quality of life during the five months of chemotherapy that I had to endure.

7

Movement Is Medicine

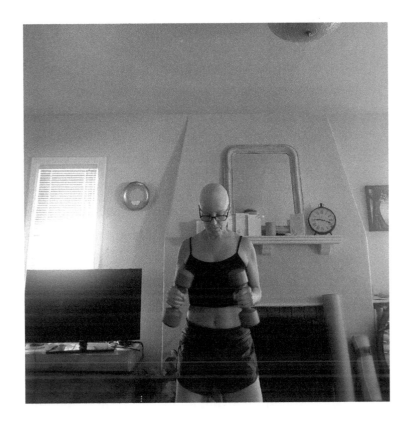

Naturally, I love to exercise. For most of my life, I have exercised or did some kind of movement every single day.

When I talked to my entire care team, I was informed that the best thing I could do during my entire cancer journey is move. Even if it's for five to ten minutes every few hours. This was music to my ears. I thought that possibly they may tell me to just lie low and heal.

Since I had lost about 10 pounds from eating extremely healthfully through my cancer adventure, I started to wonder: What if I could rock a sexy bod right out of my cancer treatments? I planted this wish in my head. I mean, who even thinks about this during cancer treatments? Most cancer patients I knew were just trying to get through it and here I am submitting my request to the universe for six-pack abs. But you know what? Why the fuck NOT? Who is gonna stop me? So, I just went for it. I exercised all the way through my journey. Sure, there were days that I could barely get up. I would have crazy fatigue. But on those days, I would just go for walks around the block with my neighbor.

When you have that many toxins dumped into your body, you've got to sweat it out. Get that blood flow and fresh oxygen to those cells! Whenever I worked out, I never regretted it. Movement gave me more energy, less brain fog and I felt less toxic. I would dance around my living room, go for short and long walks and hike up in the redwoods. I did yoga, tai chi, online dance classes, HIIT and some resistance band workouts. I wasn't going for big muscles; I just didn't want to lose the endurance I had worked for most of my life. I wanted to detoxify and increase my energy.

A good friend of mine also brought me a mini trampoline to jump on. I had never really worked out on a trampoline before but many times I would crank up the music on my headphones and jump around for as long as I could. I was amazed at how many times I could go for 30 minutes or more even during the chemotherapy days.

Whenever I exercised, I generally felt way better and totally motivated. I was far from my usual endurance, but I was pleased when I could comfortably jump around for 20 minutes or more. My goal was to not have to start from scratch when I completed treatments. In the end, I wanted to look like a normal healthy human, not someone who had endured nine months of brutal cancer treatments.

8

Adventures
in Chemotherapy

*"If your path demands you to walk through
hell, walk as if you own the place."*
—Gaurav Singh

Just 10 days after surgery, I was scheduled for my first chemo infusion.

How in the heck do you reckon with having a metric fuckton of toxins dumped into your body knowing you may end up barfing your guts out, losing your hair and all of your feminine features, sleeping your days away, losing toenails, and dealing with mouth sores amongst so many other stupid side effects? Maybe it will happen? Maybe not. I decided once I walked through those doors that I would just turn my light up to 11 and pray that my illumination would protect me from the hell I was about to experience.

After fully grasping what may or may not happen during chemotherapy, I decided just to accept all possible outcomes: Plan for the worst and hope for the best. Although I was aware that the chemotherapy could be destructive to healthy tissues, I decided to change that belief. I chose to believe that the chemotherapy was medicine. I chose to believe that chemo would erase all the bad things in my body. I chose to believe that this process would wipe the slate clean so that I could start fresh. I thought of it like burning down a forest and later planting new trees. In the end, this thought process was instrumental in my healing.

So that I wouldn't have to be alone after chemotherapy, Ryan decided he would stay with me every night until we felt it was okay for him to go home. It was now summertime, and we made sure I was well equipped with portable air conditioners for the bedroom and living room in case of heat waves. This ended up being a lifesaver as we had both heat waves and tons of wildfires surrounding the Bay Area.

I was told by my nurse navigator and other breast cancer survivors who had received the same treatment I was prescribed that the first two months are the worst because they initially hit you with the hardest, most aggressive drugs called AC, which is a combination of two chemotherapy drugs used to treat breast cancer. The initials stand for Adriamycin (also called doxorubicin) and cyclophosphamide. Many breast cancer survivors call it the Red Devil. The drug has a red color and, once administered, causes you to pee red for up to two days. AC is so strong that the drugs can only be administered every other week. The inner five-year-old in me was super excited about peeing colors. I also knew that the more water that I drank, the faster I could move that color out. I also could tell that I was hydrating myself well if the red disappeared by that evening.

I did much research about reducing the abusive side effects of chemotherapy and one thing that consistently came up was fasting. Fasting means to not eat or take any supplementation and just drink water. The typical protocol for fasting during chemo is to fast the day before treatment, the day of, and the day after. Many of the women who fasted reported that they didn't have any nausea or vomiting on the days following chemo treatment. Some reported having more energy as well. Studies posted on the National Center for Biotechnology Information's website shows that short-term fasting protects healthy cells against the adverse effects of chemotherapy while making tumor cells more vulnerable, by aggressively attacking the tumor plus reducing side effects. Well, that sounded like a winner. So the day before chemotherapy I decided to go ahead and fast.

I'll admit, I was both anxious and curious about how chemotherapy day would go, which meant I didn't sleep all that well the night before. I kept thinking, "You really don't know your own strength until you are literally forced to jump off of the cliff." I felt like I was free falling into a hole of uncertainty. We had no idea what exactly was going to happen to me. Would I have a reaction? Would I be puking my guts out for days? Would I sleep for days? Or would this kill me instantly? We just didn't know.

Knowing that I would be hanging out at the cancer center for several hours, I decided to arm myself with fun projects. I packed color and sketch books, music, my computer, and two water bottles. Forty-five minutes prior to my appointment, I had to apply lidocaine cream on my skin over the port where they inject the drugs. I applied that shit like thick frosting so that I wouldn't feel a damn thing.

My girlfriends came over and cleaned my house from top to bottom so that every speck of dust, dirt, and mold was accounted for so that it wouldn't make me sick. Knowing I had a clean house to come home felt really nice too!

Due to COVID restrictions, Ryan wasn't allowed to come inside with me, so he dropped me off in front of the cancer center. As he opened the car door at the curb and helped me gather the last of my things, we hugged each other really tight. Both of us were anxious about the quantities of toxins being dumped into my body and how I would respond.

Because my nurse navigator warned us that it wasn't a good idea to make out for a few days after chemo, we decided to put on a show in the parking lot. We stuck our tongues out, slobbering on each other's faces, making that noise a baby makes when they discover they can make noises with their tongues. I'm sure it was quite a scene amongst all of the sick people making their way into the cancer center.

I walked in; head held high armed with enough lidocaine on my port area to numb the entire upper half of my body. I checked in and waited in my invisible suit of armor. Chemo, let's get one thing straight: You and I are gonna duke it out hard and let's just be clear. I'm going to come out with the winning trophy.

"Ellen Olson!!!" the nurse called out.

Okay, it's game time. She took all my vitals and escorted me to the infusion room.

My first sight of the infusion space wasn't at all what I expected. It was a very large space with private rooms with bathrooms and sliding glass doors. Those rooms were arranged along the outer areas of the space. The nurses' station sat in the middle for easy access.

The room I was escorted to was about 10 X 10, filled with equipment and a green reclining chair. There were pictures on the wall drawn by a child—rainbows, sunshine, and stick figures with the words, "Hope you get well soon!" This filled me with so much love it brought me to tears. I got myself settled into the reclining heated chair and anxiously waited for what was next. A young man came in and offered me a heated blanket which was a nice touch! Luxurious perks already.

My oncology nurse arrived and explained to me how chemo day would go down. First, we needed to do a few blood tests. Blood tests were reviewed by my oncologist, who would give the thumbs up to start treatment if everything looked good. Before administering AC, she would give me a few support drugs, as well as saline for hydration: dexamethasone (a steroid to help reduce nausea, fatigue and inflammation) and a cocktail of anti-nausea medications. All of these medications were given intravenously through my port.

The nurse admired my fabulously thorough lidocaine application around the port area. There was no way in hell I wanted to feel any needles piercing into the right side of my tiny cleavage. She prepped the area and counted to three. I sat, waiting to feel something but that sucker was already in! She was smooth! The needle has a long tube attached to it, where she can draw blood and also administer medications. As much as I hated my port, I did see the value in having it. Otherwise, I wouldn't be able to draw or type. It would have been difficult to go to the bathroom AND I wouldn't have to get stabbed by needles so often.

Now that she had access to my port, blood was drawn for white and red counts, glucose, kidney and liver function, platelets, sodium, potassium, and so on. AND a pregnancy test every single time. Ugh. Who would want to get pregnant through this? I was certainly not thinking of being in the throes of passion while my head is in the toilet.

About 30 minutes later, the blood counts came up with a red flag. My glucose levels were too low to administer the meds! I guess fasting before chemo wasn't such a good idea after all! My oncologist paid me a visit to find out just what the heck was going on. I explained to her all my research on fasting. She wasn't aware that this was even a thing! She told me if my glucose levels were too low then they could not begin treatment. I was handed a pack of saltine crackers to get my glucose up.

In the meantime, Reggie pulled rank and decided to come meet me for most of my chemo session. She also happened to know a few of the ladies who worked in the cancer center. I spent the next four hours chatting and laughing with Reggie as a few of the staff popped their heads in to say hi. Reggie had asked them to check on me, but because she was also there, the room became filled with laughter and it was almost as if I had forgotten why I was even there in the first place. This was probably the most socializing I had done since the pandemic started three months ago!

When it was time to start the chemo drugs, my oncology nurse showed up in Tyvek and eye protection to administer my chemotherapy. These drugs are so toxic that if you so much as get one tiny drop on you, it could make you sick. Especially for anyone exposed to it daily!

She slowly injected the Adriamycin into the line that went straight to my port. The entire process of administering this drug took about 30 minutes total. Once finished, she hung the bag of cyclophosphamide and attached it to my port line. After about 90 minutes, I was finished.

Before I could leave, my oncology nurse applied a small rectangular patch to my right lower abdomen. This patch had a timer on it that would automatically administer the drug Neulasta, which is a white-blood-cell booster. A side effect of many chemotherapy drugs is that it lowers white blood counts. Neulasta would help keep my white counts at a healthy level. Once she applied the patch, within about 30 seconds I simultaneously heard a snapping sound and a pin prick to my skin. The needle had inserted itself into my abdomen for the drug to be administered at 9 p.m. the next day. This should be interesting.

I texted Ryan to let him know I was ready to be picked up. When he arrived, I walked toward the car with my sunglasses on and a smile on my face. He looked somewhat confused by all of this. I know he wasn't sure what to expect, but he did think that I'd either be wheeled to the car in a wheelchair, drooling with a puke bowl in my lap or that I'd be walking out slow and unsteady.

I didn't get home until about 6 p.m. that night. At that point, I was hungry but felt weird. Oddly, I craved deep-fried tater tots. It was a rare thing for me to ever want something deep fried but Ryan ordered tater tots to be delivered just to be sure I would eat something.

I was armed with two different types of anti-nausea pills plus steroids to take for three days after treatment.

I knew the steroids that were given to me through my IV would keep me awake all night, so I made a list of projects that I wanted to complete. I decided that instead of being frustrated about not sleeping, I would take advantage of this opportunity to accomplish something. For all I knew, I might not feel so hot the next day. I spent all night building my new online sales website and watched a few episodes of *Schitt's Creek*. I finally began to pass out around 6 a.m. and was awakened by the loud ringtone on my phone. It was Reggie checking in on me to see how I was doing. She also wanted to make sure I had a bowel movement since Zofran, the anti-nausea medicine, can turn your poops into bricks. I was proud to report to Reggie that the big number two happened right after I got home from chemotherapy! Gold stars all around for this chick!

I had mentally prepared myself for the worst, but I never did feel sick. I actually felt hyper-focused and energized from the steroids. The day after my first chemotherapy, I organized one of my closets and jumped on the reformer for a little while to burn off the excess energy.

I felt a little off but totally functional. It was like the drugs gave me magic powers. I wanted to organize everything and take on tedious projects that I would normally procrastinate doing otherwise.

Ryan was so relieved that I was responding so well. He was still working and taking meetings all day. He was grateful that he didn't have to hold my hair while I was throwing up or help me get around the house. I felt okay. Not 100%. But not terrible.

The only thing that we weren't sure about was this white blood booster patch that was attached to my stomach. It was supposed to inject meds around 9 p.m. that night. What could go wrong? This was supposed to give a boost to my immune system, right? I felt like it was okay to send him home. Though I felt a little weird, I had felt way worse from previous years when I ended up with a nasty flu bug or cold. I said, "Go home and rest. This is gonna inject meds to boost my white blood counts. How horrible can that be?" Honestly, I wanted him to go home and so he wouldn't be on my case for spontaneously spring cleaning or tearing apart my bedroom closet.

Reluctant to leave, he packed up his overnight bag and headed back to his place just 30 minutes away.

He said, "If you have any problems you call me right away. Okay, Bean?"

"Okay, Squeaks." Squeaks is my nickname for him and to entertain your curiosity, this name came about because he makes weird squeaky sounds when he sleeps.

I was feeling a bit tired after he left so I decided to lie on the couch and binge watch *Schitt's Creek*. At some point, I had passed out face down. During the time I was sleeping, the Neulasta patch had already administered the drug. Around 9:30 p.m. I woke up with my face stuffed in a pillow, feeling extremely nauseated. I decided to grab a bowl from the kitchen to sit next to me on the couch as I refused to lie waiting on the bathroom floor for something to happen. As soon as I stood up, I felt hot and dizzy, as if an energetic weight was pushing me down. I reached for the wall in the dining room and that's the last thing I remember.

I woke up underneath the dining table dripping with sweat. Why am I under the table? I should probably get up but this cold floor feels so good! This is absurd! You need to get off the floor!

And then the unbearable cramping in my stomach began. What the fuck is happening? Afraid to stand up, I crawled out from under the dining room table to my couch. Oh no. I don't want to call Ryan and tell him that I somehow ended up under the dining room table. He just got home! I'm sure I'm fine! But as sweat began dripping and the painful cramping fired up, I changed my mind. Once I could focus again and talked myself through how to use my phone, I successfully got a ring tone.

"Hey Bean."

Me: "Please don't panic. I think I fainted when I got up off the couch and ended up under the dining table."

Ryan: "Are you okay? Did you hit your head?"

Me: "I must have. I don't know. I don't remember."

Ryan: "Okay, I'm on my way."

Not more than one minute later, my neighbor Nara came knocking on my door. Ryan had called her to check up on me. "Hey, are you okay? Can you let me in?"

I lay there on the couch, unable to get my legs to work.

"I can't!" I mumbled.

"Ellen, are you in there? Are you okay? Can you let me in?"

I gave myself the biggest pep talk. You can do this. All you gotta do is stand up. Slowly, I stood up, holding on to the couch with every step I made towards the door and I let her in. Victory!!! I made it back to the couch, sweating with intense cramping.

I was in my underwear and t-shirt, sweating profusely and apologized for being smelly. I couldn't shower until the Neulasta patch had administered the meds and that I could safely take it off.

Nara mentioned the lovely knot on my forehead. I couldn't even feel it. She asked how many fingers she was holding up and kept chatting with me to see if I had any signs of a concussion. I was making complete sense and wasn't slurring so that was a plus. All signs pointed to no concussion.

I didn't want to talk and so she did some light massage to my lower legs and feet until Ryan arrived. This was so calming that the cramping subsided and I felt more relaxed. It wasn't too long after Nara arrived that Ryan showed up, a bit panicked and noticing the goose-egg lump on my forehead. Surprisingly, it did not hurt. After I had calmed down and stopped sweating, sat up, and chatted with them both, it appeared I was okay. We all decided that a visit to the emergency wasn't necessary. After all, that's the last place we wanted to be during the pandemic.

To be extra cautious, Ryan decided that he would set his alarm clock hourly to check in on me all night long to make sure I was okay. I was not happy about it. I mean, I got it, but I was just so tired after being up all night and not sleeping at all during the day. I decided to sleep on the couch instead of sleeping in my bed. At the time, I had a large captain's bed that was about four feet high. The last thing I needed was to fall out of bed if I had to use the bathroom. That night, every hour, Ryan got out of bed to wake me up to see if I was still alive. I was super grumpy about it, but glad he did. I made it through the night with no issues.

The next day, I contacted my nurse navigator, and she went through a checklist of questions to make sure that I didn't have any signs of a concussion. Thankfully, the bump on my head had shrunk and I never once had a headache. I did, however, end up with a nice bruise as a badge of chemo-related injury. She also informed me that it was not uncommon to have weird reactions to the Neulasta patch the very first time and that generally after that, it would be smooth sailing.

I'm so grateful that it wasn't worse. This was probably the worst thing that happened to me during all of my five months of chemotherapy.

The second worst thing was the time I had what I call brick turds. Any cancer patient taking anti-nausea medication must get very comfortable discussing bowel movements with their oncologist and nurses. Anyone who knows me understands that I have no issues with this. Maybe it's because my parents rewarded me so well each time I successfully pooped in the potty. Pooping is awesome. I mean, it's kinda gross and all BUT it's always a relief to go, right? No one likes to feel bloated. If we've met, and I think you're cool, it will only be a matter of time before I talk to you about pooping. Heck, if I fart in front of you this means we have a real connection. I'm the real deal with human bodily functions just like everyone else. The only difference is, I'm more vocal about it.

One of the side effects of taking these anti-nausea meds is constipation or what I like to call brick turds. Brick turds are exactly what it sounds like—super large, hard stools that are difficult to pass. Even though I was eating a healthy diet and I focused on eating lots of fiber, I ended up having excruciating brick turds. I drank Smooth Move tea to help and while it helped a little, it wasn't the stool softener that I needed. If I had known what I know now, I would have begun taking laxatives and stool softeners from the very beginning.

For the first month of chemotherapy, I did all right in the pooping department. The next month, not so much. It was so awful, I ended up with painful fissures that came and went even several months after I was finished with chemotherapy.

I struggled terribly one time for about a week. The gentle laxatives and teas were not working. Ryan was so worried that he hit up the pharmacy and damn near cleared their shelves of every laxative and enema in stock. I wasn't allowed to use any enemas or suppositories without consent from my doctor. But there was no other alternative—ol' brick turd was NOT coming out without assistance.

I contacted my nurse navigator, desperate for a solution. After she discussed it with my oncologist, she called me back with thumbs-up for suppositories and called it into my pharmacy. Ryan, tired of feeling constipated from my constipation, raced over to the pharmacy and picked them up for me. We read the instructions on the package to make sure I knew what I was getting myself into. We were excited to learn that this would soften the stool and evacuate brick turd within 20 to 30 minutes. I popped that sucker into my suffering booty hole and waited.

At the time, I lived in a cute little one-bedroom cottage. Ryan thought that going out for a walk to give me some privacy would be a good idea. I was so glad he did. On that hot August day, I gave birth to brick turd around 6 p.m., letting out a shriek of both terror and joy. And that box lied. No softening happened to that poo. I looked down at brick turd and prayed to God that it would actually flush.

About 10 minutes after I recovered from the most terrifying shit of my life, Ryan walked in the door to see me seated on the couch. He looked at me like "well?" I said, "It happened!" He ran to me and hugged me with such excitement and then began pacing the living room.

"OH MY GOD! I HAVE TO WORRY ABOUT HOW YOU ARE GONNA SURVIVE EACH AND EVERY CHEMO TREATMENT AND NOW I HAVE TO WORRY ABOUT YOUR SHITS?!!!" And then we both burst into laughter. Real love is when you don't have to feel insecure about basic human bodily functions. I felt so lucky that I had a partner I could be 100% myself with. Even when it's crappy. No pun intended.

Throughout my AC treatments, I did pretty well. It wasn't enjoyable, but I survived it well. I never once vomited. I did experience fatigue. Once I had finished taking my steroids three days after my infusions, I had to do hard-core napping for about three days. My infusions were every other week on Tuesdays. Wednesday through Friday, the steroids gave me super energy powers. Saturday through Monday, I had brain fog and would nap off and on throughout the day. On occasion, I would get heartburn. Ginger tea worked like a charm.

My nails started looking strange. They had more ridges and got very thick on the tips. One of my middle toenails turned black and blue. It stayed that way for about a month after I completed chemo and fell off. But there was already a fresh new nail underneath. On occasion, I would get mouth sores and would rinse a few times a day with water and baking soda, which did the trick. My teeth looked as if they were cracking and turned grey. I found it hard to eat crunchy foods. Staying hydrated was a full-time job. I was drinking somewhere around 100 ounces or more per day. My skin felt dry and scaly so I slathered oil on my skin as much as I could.

For me, AC did a number on my cognitive function. I became forgetful and had a difficult time completing tasks. I had check-off lists for just getting out the door and had to set up reminders in my calendar for my daily self-care. I had difficulty being present for conversations. I had a hard time holding space to listen. Talking was a chore. I would forget what I was talking about mid-sentence.

My digestion felt sluggish. Sometimes I would lose my appetite for a few days. I craved foods I wouldn't usually eat. I love vegetables but hated the idea of eating cooked veggies. I really wanted a salad but because my white counts were low, I was advised not to eat raw veggies because the risk of bacterial infections was too high. Eventually, my taste buds stopped working and everything started to taste bland.

Because I was doing chemotherapy during a pandemic and we were all ordered to stay home, I treated my chemo sessions like my social time. I had a chance to be around other people! And as my nurses slowly administered the Adriamycin, this was an opportunity to chat and get to know each other.

I also brought a list of things I wanted to accomplish during chemotherapy. Maybe it was to do some drawing or coloring. Some days I would work on my business plan or finish designing my website. I spent a lot of time writing newsletters too.

I'm also very playful and ridiculously silly. So why not bring that part of myself into my cancer treatments? I love dressing up in costumes and being in character. On my second AC treatment, I showed up with fake teeth and a shirt that resembled a shirtless hairy man. The nipples and hairy chest were totally disgusting and even more so on a woman. My friend Jodi told me once, "Ellen, you're the only woman I know that loves to look scary." It kept a lot of men from bothering me. People's reactions are always hysterical. I felt like the nurses in oncology could use a chuckle after dealing with life threatening illnesses all day long.

On several occasions I wore light-up kitty-ear headphones, whacky leggings and giant, pink monster feet. One patient who sat near me loved them.

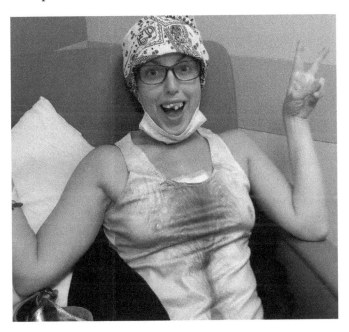

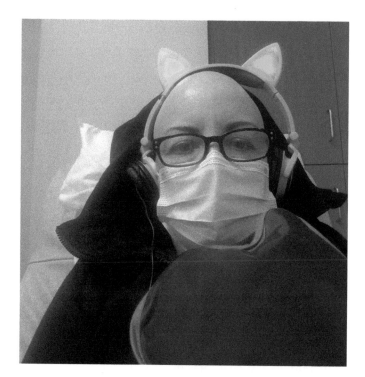

I did want to respect other people's experience at the cancer center. Cancer is no joke. But humor was a slice of heaven for me that brought me joy and gave me fuel to press on. And the patients that got to see me—well, it gave them a chuckle too.

The AC treatments felt like an eternity. But the lump in my breast and lymph nodes felt as if they were dramatically reduced.

One week after my last AC infusion, I met with my surgeon for an ultrasound to find out the details of tumor shrinkage. Ryan and I talked about what the results might be and we both guessed that the tumors may have shrunk by about 25%. If we received that number, we agreed we'd feel pretty good about that.

We were still dealing with restrictions due to the pandemic, so Ryan attended my appointments through video calls. As my surgeon performed the ultrasound, I could see the difference in the tumors. At the time of my original diagnosis, there were four lymph nodes showing cancer. On this very day, just two months later, only two lymph nodes were showing up. After taking measurements of the lymph nodes and breast tumor and comparing against the original measurements, we discovered that the cancer had been reduced by 48%. We weren't expecting that number. Ryan kept asking my surgeon the dimensions of the tumor just to make sure.

One the other side of the camera, my surgeon and I were jumping for joy. But Ryan was on the other side trying to calculate the dimensions to understand just how much the tumor had shrunk. She said, "Ryan!!! This is great news!! Ellen is responding well to treatment!!!"

He went silent. I couldn't tell if he was just trying to keep his cool or if he was in shock. I said, "Okay, sweetie, I'm going to get dressed and will call you in a bit."

I practically skipped all the way out to my car, calling my parents to deliver the good news.

When I made it home, I called Ryan to ask him if he was okay. I couldn't tell what was happening for him during our video call. "Hey, Squeaks! Oh my God, Can you believe it?" I shrieked.

"Bean, do you know what this means? Your tumors shrunk by almost 50%! I set up a spreadsheet to calculate the tumor reduction, but I only set up the calculations for around 30%. So I had to recalibrate everything. Once I looked at the numbers and realized how much they had shrunk, I said a prayer and then had a good cry."

"Of course, you made a spreadsheet!" I just wanted to hug him so hard at that moment. We took a moment to really marinate in this good news and once we hung up, I made a celebratory post to my cheer squad.

I wasn't done yet. I still had to do 12 more weeks of chemotherapy. My treatments were being switched to 12 weeks of Taxol, but every three weeks I would receive another drug with it called carboplatin. Because the cancer was so aggressive in the initial diagnosis, my oncologist didn't want to give it a light slap. She wanted to punch it straight out of my left side.

I heard from many cancer survivors that Taxol was a dream compared to AC. But now, my chemotherapy appointments were weekly instead of every other week. My medical team explained to me that most people don't experience nausea during Taxol, but on the days I had to receive carboplatin, I would receive anti-nausea meds in my infusions. Without Zofran, the killer anti-nausea medication, I would be sick. At one point, I asked my oncologist if she would consider using a different, less constipating anti-nausea medication. I regretted that. I was up all night with severe nausea. Though I never did throw up, I felt terrible. I decided that since I would only have to endure just three more carboplatin treatments after that, I would just beef up my laxatives. I never had to take any anti-nausea medications orally after receiving carboplatin. I seemed to only need it during my infusion. After that, it was a cake walk.

One of the side effects of Taxol is neuropathy to the hands and feet. To eliminate or drastically reduce risk of neuropathy, my medical team recommended that I purchase slip-on booties and gloves that have gel inserts that you freeze prior to wearing. My oncology nurse would alert me about five to 10 minutes before administering Taxol to slip on my cold gloves and booties. I would wear them for the duration of the Taxol drip for about an hour. Now, to add insult to injury, just before beginning Taxol, each time steroids were administered as well as a donkey punch of Benadryl straight to the brain. That Benadryl always hit me hard causing me to have restless legs. I felt my eyes rolling around like a raver in a cuddle puddle on ecstasy. I don't like being cold. What made it worse was that I was awake from the steroids, but my eyelids were heavy from the

Benadryl and my legs felt mildly electrocuted. I was on sensation overload from this experience and this ride lasted One. Whole. Hour!

I did my best to make the most out of this time by listening to audio books, watching hilarious or inspirational videos on YouTube. I tried to meditate with relaxing music, hoping I could get my mind off turning my feet and hands into a human Popsicle, but I don't think I was evolved enough to keep my mind off of being cold. I even tried to imagine myself on a tropical beach with cold coconut drinks in my hands but because I was so antsy from the Benadryl/steroid cocktail, that visualization never lasted. Sometimes I was lucky enough to be visited by one of the staff members and that made a world of difference. Chatting my way through it was the best distraction and made that hour go by quickly. When I began my Taxol/carboplatin regimen, in addition to the pandemic, the entire state of California was on fire. For several weeks, everyone was confined to their homes due to the horrible air quality. It totally sucked to be amidst our beautiful Indian summer in the middle of a pandemic and not be able to go outdoors. My walks to the beach and around the neighborhood gave me life. So I needed to find other ways to get my cardiovascular exercise. Thank goodness for YouTube! There are tons of interesting and fun dance and yoga classes. I would also turn on some house music and dance around my house. Other times, I would send videos to my friends and family of me singing karaoke and dancing round in glittery costumes and ridiculous outfits. I also would step into my alter ego, the Great Baldini, and give fortune readings. Now don't get me wrong, there were many days that my energy would only allow for me to lie around and binge watch Netflix.

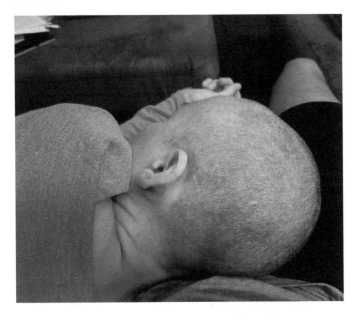

When I was just too tired to even lift a finger, I just allowed myself the space to rest. I would lie on my PEMF mat and listen to ambient sounds or audio books. I would read. I would nap. I reminded my busy, squirrely self that it was okay to take this time to heal. Sitting still is really tough for me. I always felt like I needed to be doing something. But truthfully, I believe that the cancer came here to teach me a lesson in doing nothing. It's okay to do absolutely nothing. No one should ever feel guilt or shame for not showering all day, lounging in pajamas all day, ordering in food and chilling the fuck out! Prior to cancer, I would habitually shame myself for having days like this; now I understand how important these days are for basic survival and I celebrate my down time. I find that I actually get more accomplished when I allow myself the time to rejuvenate.

Another interesting thing that Taxol can do is really mess with your tastebuds. During AC I craved greasy, fried foods and milkshakes. And while I did my best not to eat those things, I allowed myself to indulge on occasion when my appetite wasn't allowing for anything else.

With Taxol, I craved very sweet, tart foods. If it weren't for the high risk of getting mouth sores and indigestion, I would have sucked on lemons all day. Instead, I made big batches of healthy lemon bars and kept them in the fridge for a nice, cold tart dessert. I ate tart cherries, grapes, berries, and apples throughout my entire Taxol treatment. I would bring bags of grapes to chemotherapy.

I learned from a lot of cancer survivors and my medical team that weight gain through Taxol was a big concern. On average, I found that a lot of women finished their Taxol treatments with an extra 20 or more pounds. My sweet tooth tried to strong-arm me into eating tart sorbets and vanilla ice cream with raspberries and sweet syrups, but I was not okay with gaining weight. After all, I wasn't in the financial position to buy new clothes. I worked hard enough to stay alive during chemotherapy and the last thing I wanted was to work hard at losing weight. I also knew that when I made healthier choices, my body responded better to treatments and I didn't feel so crappy. I enjoyed eating fresh, tart fruits and allowed myself the occasional sweet dessert from time to time. I gained a total of five pounds in my 12 weeks of the Taxol/carboplatin regimen, which disappeared after one month of getting back to my regular healthy eating habits.

There were three occasions where my port decided to flip on its side. I was concerned about this after it was surgically implanted. I am active and do a lot of different exercises. I stayed active throughout chemotherapy. I'm also an active sleeper and at times would wake up on my stomach with a pile of pillows on top of me. I'd also find myself positioned sideways, across the middle of the bed.

One Saturday morning, after I was feeling like I was recovering well from my third AC treatment and wanted to head out for a walk, I decided to get some stretching in and noticed that my chest felt tight and sore when I tried interlocking my fingers behind me to stretch out my arms and chest.

I ran to the bathroom to look in the mirror to see that it appeared that my port had flipped sideways.

Bloody hell. It looked like a tiny alien trying to escape from my chest. What the fuck am I supposed to do about this on a Saturday?

I contacted the cancer center, which was closed, but there was an oncologist on call that day. I left a detailed message about waking up to my port flipped sideways in my chest and about 30 minutes the on-call oncologist called me back. I was hoping I could walk in and someone could flip it back for me. But nope, this was a job for my surgeon.

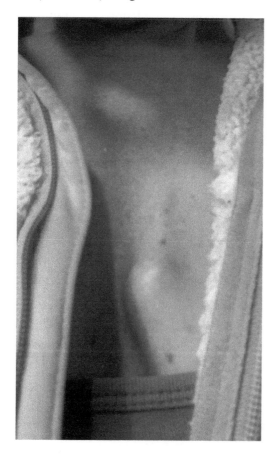

I called my surgeon's office, which was also closed. Thankfully, there was a surgeon on call who contacted me back. She walked me through some steps on how to maneuver it back into place but it was super painful. That port was wedged into my cleavage sideways and I could not get it to budge. She said, "I don't have anyone available to flip this for you today, but if you'd like to come in on Monday morning at 8 a.m., I can flip it for you. If it's too painful and you want to get this done now, you can go to the emergency room and they may be able to find someone to flip it back for you." Since this was not life-threatening AND it was uncomfortable, not painful, I decided to just wait until Monday. I was definitely not waiting for hours in the midst of a pandemic to get this port flipped. I would spare myself the insanity, thank you very much.

On Monday morning, Ryan drove me to the surgeon's office. We fully intended that I might be in pain when she was finished. She took one look at it and confirmed that it had indeed flipped on its side. I was nervous; I had no idea how much she would need to manhandle it to move back into place. She laid me back on the table and tilted the table backwards a bit so that my head was practically in her lap. She worked it in her fingers back and forth a bit and in less than 60 seconds, that sucker painlessly snapped right back into place! I damn near skipped out of her office! I called Ryan, who was waiting in the car in a parking lot. He was so surprised that she was done quickly and, more important, that I wasn't in any pain whatsoever. In fact, when I got home, I walked straight to the beach for a three-and-a-half mile walk.

About six weeks later, my port flipped again. Only this time it flipped completely upside down. I was having a horrible time that week. My blood counts had dropped, I was tired, and struggling with painful fissures that weren't healing from that monstrosity brick turd I gave birth to weeks ago.

I was fed up with chemotherapy at this point and now, my damn port had flipped again. My surgeon attempted to flip it but it was so painful I let out a shriek and began to cry. I completely lost it. She was so incredibly compassionate. I'll admit, prior to my cancer diagnosis, my experience with western doctors left me feeling pretty hopeless about healthcare. She pulled out the Kleenex box and validated every thought in my mind. She reminded me that no matter how strong you are, that the cancer journey is very difficult and that it was okay to feel all of what I was feeling. I needed that.

Once I had regrouped, she decided to schedule me for an in-office procedure. She would have to make an incision to flip the port and then suture me back up. Before doing this procedure, she had to see where my blood counts were. Unfortunately, my platelets and white blood counts had dropped so low that my risk of infection was high. I had seven Taxol treatments to go and we didn't want to do anything so risky that could potentially interfere with my treatments. Instead, at Ryan's suggestion, she injected the area with lidocaine and after a lot of manipulating, she flipped that port back into place with minimal discomfort.

I thought I was to blame for the port shifting but this wasn't entirely the case. My surgeon explained to me that she sutures the port in place so that it wouldn't move, but apparently my sutures dissolved, and this baby was free floating in my chest area.

With just seven weeks of chemotherapy left, I did my best to sleep on my back and use pillows to keep me from sleeping on my stomach. One week before I was finished with chemo, the port flipped sideways again. I was so frustrated and filled with rage. I was so out of fucks at that point that I leaned forward, using gravity to help me move it back into place. And like a total savage, I successfully, for the last time, flipped that bitch like a boss.

The only other bump in the road I was faced with during my Taxol/carboplatin treatments was my plummeting drop in red and white blood counts. To address my white counts, I was prescribed Zarxio, which was a shot that I had to administer subcutaneously into my abdomen. With everything else I had to endure, giving myself a shot in the gut three to four days a week was nothing.

At one point, my hemoglobin (red counts) had dropped to 6.7. Healthy hemoglobin needs to read at about 11.7. This is a normal thing that happens during chemotherapy. However, my medical team was a bit stumped by my energy and how healthy I appeared. Various nurses came in and asked how I was feeling. By no stretch did I feel "normal," but I was in good spirits and had done a 30-minute cardio dance workout prior to showing up for chemotherapy. Each new person that walked in to check on me just couldn't understand where my energy was coming from.

"What are you doing?" they asked.

"I get high-dose Vitamin C infusions weekly, acupuncture weekly, do moxibustion at least four days a week, eat a healthy diet, meditate on my PEMF/infrared mat, exercise and take a long list of supplements to support me through treatments." I said.

"Well, it is obviously working because you are doing so good!"

I could feel just how much their minds were blown. And this, my friends, is exactly why it was important for me to do as many holistic treatments as I could do.

In the last few weeks leading up to my last day of chemotherapy, I decided that I wanted to throw some kind of a party in celebration of finishing chemo and to also thank the entire staff for their amazing care and compassion. They helped me turn something so frightening to me into a positive experience. I made beautiful connections with these ladies and it was bittersweet to be finishing. While I was excited to end this chapter of my journey, I was also sad not to see their faces on the regular. Each of the staff was so wonderful and they deserved recognition.

One day, when I showed up for treatment, I was taken to this incredibly large room with a big picture window looking out into the trees that lined the street. It was a gorgeous fall day filled with blue skies and brightly colored orange and yellow leaves. Whitney, one of Reggie's friends who worked in oncology, stopped in to visit me that day and remarked that she had no idea that room was used for chemotherapy. I called it the pimp suite. I mean, I felt like I was getting VIP chemotherapy!

I had mentioned to both my nurse navigator and to Whitney that I wanted to have a karaoke dance party on my last day and that I also wanted to ring a victory bell. Whitney said, "I don't think a bell would work for you. You need a gong!"

In fact, Whitney decided to buy a gong and the day she visited me in the VIP suite, she brought a box in for me to open and inside the box was a gong for my last day of chemo! I told her that I needed to have the pimp suite for my last day karaoke dance party. I spoke to my nurse navigator also that day and she agreed that the room was perfect. It was nowhere near any other patients and big enough to have a small number of people. They also authorized Ryan to come for my last day.

The day before my last chemo treatment, I furiously baked delicious desserts to bring to the nurses. I packed my party outfit as I just didn't feel right walking into the cancer center full of sick people decked out in a rainbow sequin jumpsuit.

Ryan also put together a DJ set so I could dance around in my cold mitts and gloves.I showed up on my last day with my microphone and speaker, sequin outfit, an arsenal of baked goods, smiles and good vibes! Reggie showed up after we got settled in too!

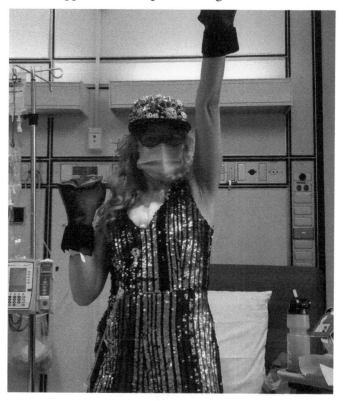

We started first thing in the morning at 8 a.m. and my last day went so quickly, I was out the door by 11 a.m.

Reggie sang the theme song from *The Golden Girls* tv sitcom, "Thank You for Being a Friend." This is a song that Reggie and our gang sang when we regularly got together. It was OUR theme song! Reggie also had to test the gong by taking a few good whacks at it.

The minute my oncology nurse removed the needle from my port, I danced and sang "Car Wash" and banged the crap outta that gong. That was the last time I would be stabbed in the chest for a while and hopefully for good.

When I was done, we packed up our things and got ready to head out. I was feeling weird about walking out in my jumpsuit in front of all of the folks in the waiting room. I wanted to respect their journey. But Elizabeth, my nurse navigator, encouraged me to wear it. So down the elevator I went, in my purple wig, sparkly jumpsuit, and ridiculous gold hat. As we stepped out into the open, Reggie yelled, "Hey everyone! It's her last day of chemo!" People cheered and clapped!

I was too energized and filled with joy to even feel tired from it all. Closing this chapter was one of the best days of my life.

9

Healthy Mindset Boot Camp

The strongest muscle and worst enemy is your mind. Train it well.

Often, we don't know or don't believe that we can heal ourselves with our minds.

Have you ever been so uncomfortably hot that you have imagined yourself inside an icy igloo? Do try it! You can actually get your body to believe that it is cold. I once turned on a YouTube video of a snowy mountainscape during a heat wave, and after a few minutes I needed a sweater!

Have you ever been able to calm your own nerves, just by focusing on being calmer?

We've all been in situations where we've been uncomfortable and have changed the conversation in our minds. Instead of thinking, "I'm so miserably hot," you can tell yourself that you are inside an igloo at the North Pole freezing your ass off. Just thinking about it can change how you feel. Or if you're ever super nervous before a presentation, you can think, "I am strong, I am powerful. People are interested in what I have to say." This can give you the courage to walk in front of your audience to make your speech.

During my entire cancer journey, these are just a few of the phrases I would say out loud daily.

"I feel incredible."

"I am a powerful healer."

"My body has the power to heal itself."

"I am filled with joy."

"I am beautiful."

"I am a brilliant light."

"Today, I honor that my body wishes to relax and heal."

"I am loved."

"I am prosperous."

"I have fun wherever I go."

"Today will be an awesome day."

"I am successful in my work today."

"My white blood counts have risen to 4.0."

"My body is free from negativity."

"From the top of my head, to the bottom of my feet, every bone, cell, tissue, fluid, and organs are strong, healthy and activated. They are shielded from all negativity."

"This juice tastes delicious!"

On the days I was afraid, I would tell myself that it was okay to be scared sometimes but reminded myself that I was indeed much bigger than my cancer and that my body possessed all the magical powers to heal. I would talk to my cells, telling them about how strong and powerful they were. I would visualize my white blood counts being at normal, healthy levels. I would play video games with my cancer almost like "Space Invaders." I would imagine myself shooting the cancer until it was completely gone. I visualized my cancer being driven out of my body by a tiny dump truck and dumped out into the universe and it would turn into stars. I saw my cells as being so active and healthy that they looked like clear glass bubbles but with the strength of a tank.

On the days I felt bad, I would remind myself that this was temporary and then visualized all that brought me joy. I imagined myself in places I hadn't visited, like riding a bike in the Swiss Alps or sitting in a warm steamy hot tub looking out onto snowy mountaintops. I would picture myself in paradise and tell myself that I would get to visit all of these places when I was done with my treatments.

I also thought about what it would feel like to help someone in need. To cheer up someone sad. I would put on a playlist that would lift me up and dance around my house. I would make goofy videos for my friends and sing karaoke to them. I would watch funny videos when I needed to laugh. I roamed the neighborhood with my neighbor in costumes and lights at night, dragging my karaoke mic and singing.

Magical things happen when you send the right messages to your mind and body.

10

Beauty and Hair Loss

"We delight in the beauty of the butterfly, but rarely admit the changes it has gone through to achieve that beauty."
—Maya Angelou

I have to admit that losing my hair on my head didn't bother me as much as losing my lashes and brows. I was a bit excited to be pushed off of this ledge and take on the challenge of going deeper into self-acceptance. I felt like losing my hair would liberate me from any stupid, bought-in beliefs around what it is to be beautiful. I truly believed that my hair wasn't what made me beautiful but instead who I am at the very core of my being. So, fuck anyone who tells me any different. At the end of the day, with or without hair, I'm still me and I like me.

Truthfully, when I saw bald women, I felt like everything that hid their face had been stripped away. I loved getting a good view of their facial structure and tone. The shape and brightness of their eyes could be seen.

Just two days before my second AC treatment, my hair began to shed way more than usual. At the time, my hair was very thick, coarse, and landed a little bit past my shoulders. Ryan and I had been out exercising that day, so I had my hair tied up in a ponytail. Later that night, I decided to let my hair down and started running my fingers through my hair and massaging my scalp, which always felt good after letting my hair down. When I pulled my fingers out, chunks of hair fell to the floor. To be sure if this was really happening, I hung my head upside down and began aggressively scratching my head and it continued to fall out in large amounts. The idea of going to bed and waking up in a pool of loose hair sounded too gross and messy. I presented the hairs to Ryan and we both agreed that it was time to shave it all off! Our curiosity had us kind of excited about what was really under all that hair. What did it look like? Are there any marks or dents on it? Is it perfectly round? Or am I a conehead? I had so much hair, it was hard to tell! Ryan grabbed his clippers and we set ourselves up in the kitchen.

Of course, for me, this was a good time to break out my inner freak and see how hideous I could make myself look in the various stages of head shaving. "I need to get my fake teeth for this! Shave my head straight down the middle so I'm bald on top and the hairs are long on the side."

Ryan could never understand my obsession with looking like a scary hillbilly. I could play the part so well. The second I put those fake teeth in, I could channel the redneck that just pulled up in his rusty Ford pickup with fresh possum killings for supper in one hand and a cold Coors in the other hand.

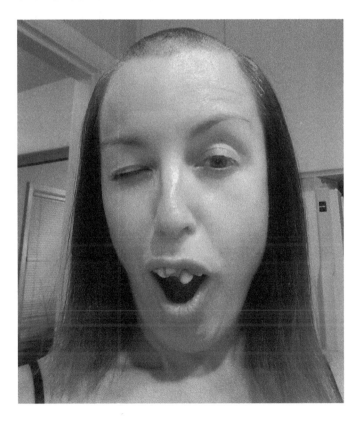

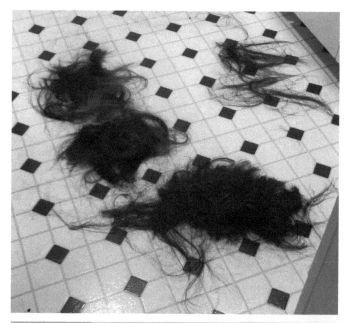

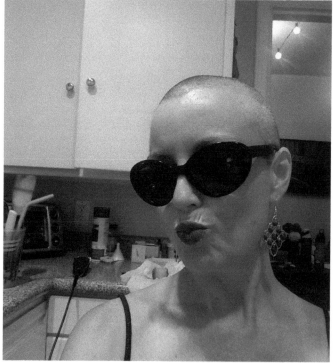

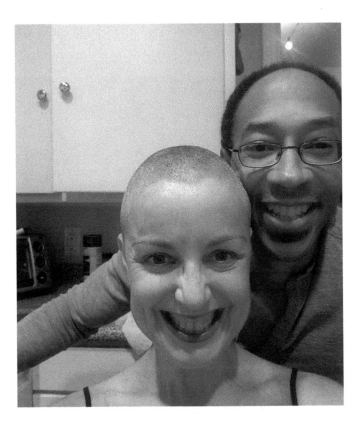

I wasn't sure if I would love my hair being shaved, but I was armed with a lot of wigs and caps in case I didn't like it. This was only temporary, and I just wanted to have fun with it.

I think it took almost an hour to get every last hair shaved off, but once we were finished, I fell in love with this new look. Without a doubt, I looked like a total badass. G.I. Jane had nothing on me.

I threw on lipstick, earrings, and sunglasses feeling like I was ready for my debut on the cover of *Vogue* magazine.

I rocked this bald look. I couldn't have cared less about the wigs now.

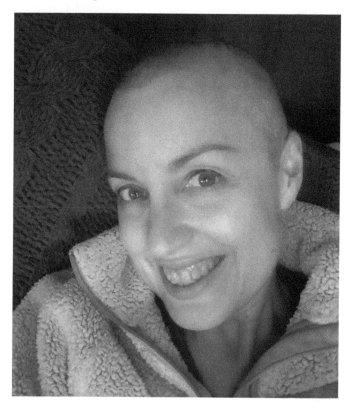

My good friend, Jodi, offered to shave her head in support, just in case I was sad about losing my hair. I wasn't sad at all. The only thing I didn't like about losing my hair was losing my brows and eyelashes. I told Jodi I could never expect her to shave her brows and pluck her lashes, so she was off the hook!

Funny enough, about the same time I shaved my head, I lost all of my pubic hair. One day, I sat down to pee and noticed a bunch of loose pubic hair in my underwear and then when I finished peeing and turned around to flush, there was pubic hair all over the toilet seat and in the toilet. It was like the scene in *A Charlie Brown Christmas* when he brings his sad tree back to the stage, sets it down on the ground and all of the needles fell off at once. THIS was exactly how I lost my pubic hair.

I jumped in the shower and managed to wash the rest of those pubes right off. This was the cheapest and most painless Brazilian wax I could have ever asked for, though I would have rather paid someone to rip my hair out. In that moment, I thought, "If someone could make a pill that would cause body hair to fall out, they would become an overnight success." I know many of my clients would have paid big money for that!

Over the course of the next several weeks, I lost every single hair on my body. Including my nostril hair. I never thought I would appreciate my nostril hair so much. Nostril hairs are like filters for our noses. They catch particles that you breathe in, preventing you from totally inhaling all the nasty stuff floating around in the air.

After I lost all of my nostril hair, my nose was constantly running and stuffy from all of the foreign objects not being filtered. For about six months, I felt like I had a perpetual cold. It would get worse every time I had a Taxol infusion. Taxol would flare up my sinuses and I was generally sneezing all night long. At that point, I understood why I was given Benadryl with each infusion!

My lashes, I found out, were also filters for my eyes. Once my lashes fell out, my eyes constantly watered until the lashes started to grow back about a month after chemo. This drove me bananas because I had purchased magnetic false eye lashes and I could hardly ever wear them because I was always wiping my runny eyes. Every now and then, I would use the lashes. Though because we were in the midst of a pandemic, there was really nowhere to really wear them.

Magnetic lashes are magic and totally safe for anyone who wants to beef up their lash game. They were so easy to apply! Just apply magnetic liquid eyeliner! Once the liner dries, then apply the magnetic strip on the liner and Voilà! You have nice, thick lashes! When I missed my girlie looks, I would pop those lashes on!

My brows were the last thing to go and I think I lost those just a couple of weeks after starting taxol. I felt like I looked like an alien without them. I would try to color them on but they always looked uneven and weird. Or I would touch my face and they would smear right off.

A friend of mind got me eyebrow stamps. The stamps came with a foam mold of an arched brow. Place the foam mold onto the brow pallet and make sure you rub it around really well to get enough brow powder on and then you stamp onto your brow area. As you can see, I had a good time with this.

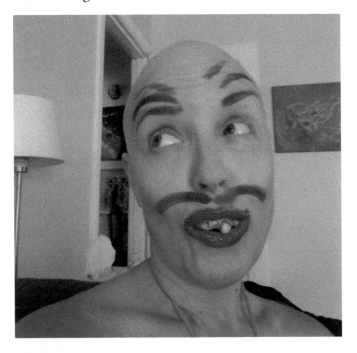

Once again, I had difficulty getting them stamped on or would somehow smear them all over my face.

And then Reggie told me about these magnificent temporary brow tattoos. Works exactly like fake tattoos! You place the tattoo over the area, saturate with water from a gauze or cotton pad for about one minute and pull the paper back. I love these because they were set up to look like individual hairs, not just one gigantic, dark line. People always complimented me on my perfect brows and how lucky I was that I had not lost my brow hair. When I told people that they were temporary tattoos, they would lose their minds! NO WAY! Plus, you could place them on your face and get them nice and straight, knowing they were in perfect position before saturating them with water. And the great thing about these: no smearing. And if you didn't rub your eyes or wash your brow area, you could stretch out their length of stay by about five days maximum.

The temporary brow tattoos were the most realistic looking and cost $20. These lasted me throughout the rest of my chemotherapy and until my brows began to grow back, which was about one month after I completed chemotherapy.

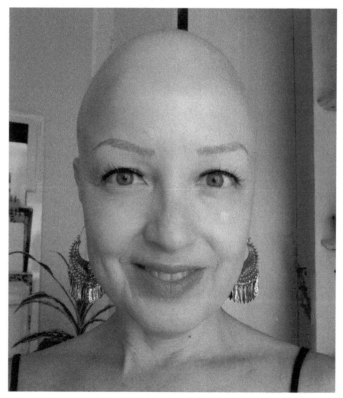

One of the other issues I had with beauty was extremely dry skin. If I put moisturizer on, my skin would be dry just minutes later. There was a cream that I used throughout my chemo and radiation treatments called Arbordoun Calendula Cream. This cream had been in my arsenal of moisturizers for the last 20 years, ever since I became an esthetician. I would use it on my clients for post-microdermabrasion or peel care. I love this cream. It's super heavy and contains so many healing and deeply moisturizing ingredients. I practically bathed in it to relieve my dry skin and later used it during my radiation treatments to keep my skin from burning. I honestly don't know what I would have done without it! I feel like it kept my skin from looking like it had aged and protected me from radiation burns.

Any time I ever felt like my vanity had been stripped away, it was nothing a pair of big, bold earrings, lipstick, giant sunglasses and a cute head scarf couldn't remedy. Besides, I wasn't going to a fancy restaurant, but there were times that I just wanted to look like a woman again. Sometimes, I just wanted to pass by the mirror and feel glamorous. The brow tattoos, lashes, lipstick, earrings, big sunglasses, and scarf or hat always did the trick!

Sometimes just putting on a cute outfit made me feel more alive and empowered. Many times, I would show up to my Vitamin C infusions and chemotherapy in cute, comfy sundresses and hats just so I could feel pretty again. Those outfits that made me feel good, vibrant and sexy, I wore them when I could. It wasn't for anyone else but me. I honestly didn't give a shit about what anyone thought about me. I dressed up for myself, if only to take a glimpse in a mirror and see the reflection of someone that didn't look like a cancer patient.

11

Post-Chemotherapy Recovery

After five months of chemo, I was completely bald, with not a hair left on any part of my body. Strangely enough, I still had a healthy glow. I had more energy than I thought I would have. Maybe it was because I was so excited to be finished or that I would be able to eat a giant salad again. Because my blood counts were low, I wasn't allowed to eat raw leafy greens. Too risky for bacterial infections that my body might have a difficult time fighting off. I couldn't wait to start getting back into my morning juicing and raw greens. I craved salads throughout all of my chemo because I went through it during a very hot summer. Eating cooked veggies didn't feel very refreshing to me at all.

Elizabeth warned me that I might be on a bit of a high after chemotherapy, but not to be surprised if over the weeks that I would feel tired and get some aches and pains. Just the chemo working itself out of my system. Because it was a full-time job for her to keep me off of my roller skates during chemo, I once again asked when it would be safe enough to start juicing again and get back on my skates. "Wait two weeks and if you aren't feeling light-headed then you can go!"

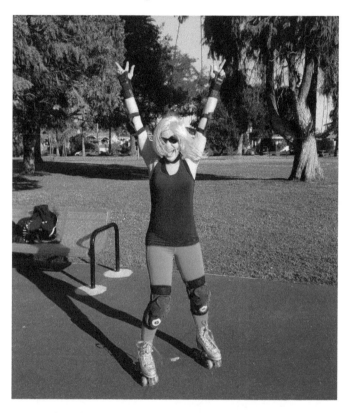

Every day during those two weeks, I made sure that I would work that chemotherapy out of my system. I lay on my PEMF mat and set my infrared settings up to high and lay under my reflective blanket to create a sauna effect. I would sweat every morning for 20 minutes. I ate extremely healthy, eating vegetable soups and making fruit protein shakes. It was important to keep the protein up for healing purposes. I would make blueberry lavender protein shakes with hemp seeds and cashew milk. I made carrot cake smoothies using cooked carrots and warm spices of ginger, clove, nutmeg, and cinnamon. I was so happy to get back into my kitchen and create yummy recipes.

Just one week after chemotherapy, I put on my running shoes and began to add some jogging into my walks. The aches and pains crept in, but I still moved. I felt sore and arthritic, but movement made me so happy, and it gave me energy.

I decided to work through my residual aches and pains by seeing my chiropractor. I was routinely seeing her every other week to keep my body in check after an injury from the previous year. I remember walking in for my very first appointment with her after I had thrown my pelvis and sacrum out. I could barely walk and was in so much pain. After receiving just one adjustment from her, I was able to walk. The pain had subsided and from then on, I saw her regularly to lower my risk of injury again.

When the pandemic hit, I had stopped going. I had no income or even time for that matter. But once I had finished chemo and felt the residual aches from chemo, I knew she could help get those aches under control.

I walked into her office and took off my cap to reveal my bald head. I just went through five months of chemo for breast cancer and I feel like an old lady. Can you make me feel young again?"

"I can fix you up, no problem. We'll get you feeling good again!"

Between her magical adjustments and the chiropractic massage therapist, within about eight weeks, I had recovered from the stiffness and aches. It no longer hurt to get out of bed. I was so excited to feel my age instead of like a 90-year-old woman!

Exactly 14 days from my last chemotherapy treatment, I got back on my skates. Because of the pandemic, all the basketball courts had their hoops removed so that people wouldn't play. Instead, these courts turned into outdoor roller rinks. I would roll out my sound system, turn up some funk, and the basketball court would come alive with other roller skaters and people dancing. This gave me life. It was so good to just feel alive and well again and to do the things I loved to do. And to also see the magic unfold around it. I felt so grateful to be able to skate under the sun, to be alive and to share this joy with others. Several of my girlfriends who skated, would mask up, dress up in wigs and costumes and meet me at the basketball court. We brought out our wireless karaoke mics, sang and skated.

I celebrated each day that I was alive. I made it through chemotherapy, one of the hardest things I had ever done in my life.

The next part of my journey was my lumpectomy. My surgeon was confident that a lumpectomy would be perfect for me as my ultrasounds weren't showing any tumors left. The only thing we could see were the metal clips where the cancer had been marked when my original biopsies were done.

My oncologist ordered a PET scan so that we could see if there was any active cancer left. PET scans give a more accurate reading of finding cancer. My video chat with my oncologist was set up 24 hours after my PET scan. A small handful of my girlfriends, who had been my big helpers during my cancer treatments and had been quarantining and getting regular COVID testing, had a get-together that day to celebrate Reggie's birthday. I wasn't sure what the news was going to be so having my girlfriends around me was comforting.

When I got on the call, I went into the bedroom where it was less noisy but everyone one by one gathered in behind me on the bed as my oncologist delivered the results. Okay, I have the results of your PET scan and you had great results. NOTHING lit up on the scan and it shows no active tumors."

I sat in disbelief as my girlfriends began shouting and celebrating behind me.

"What about the lymph nodes? Is my breast tumor gone?"

"It's all clear, Ellen."

I covered my mouth in disbelief and started laughing and crying at the same time. "Can I have my port removed when I receive my lumpectomy?"

"Yes, you can have it removed." she replied.

I'm not sure what to be more excited about, the fact that the tumors had diminished or the removal of my pain-in-the-ass port that had been doing cartwheels in my chest for the last five months.

"Thank you, Dr. G., This is the best news!!! We did it!!" I exclaimed.

Each of my girlfriends in the background thanked her for helping save my life. And even though we still had about three-and-a-half months left of treatment, I felt less afraid. We cleared up all of that cancer that had spread and now I was closer to the finish line than I was six months ago.

A few days later, I met with my surgeon to set a date and go over the details of the surgery. Ellen, your PET scan is clear! This is great news! It makes my job much easier!"

We set the date for Monday, November 30, 2020. She explained that she would be doing biopsies on my breast area and lymph nodes to make sure there was no residual cancer. Once the pathologist alerted her of any cancer cells that may be lingering, she would know what lymph nodes and any tissues that would need to be removed.

"Great job Ellen! I'll see you on the 30th!!"

After that, I contacted my parents with my surgery date. We decided that it would be nice to have them come down so that they could assist with anything I needed and also so that we could see each other. We had to do quarantining and luckily, I had to do a COVID test the weekend right before my surgery.

I took the rest of the time to strengthen and heal my body. I spent a lot of time roller skating at the basketball court and really getting it in as much as possible. I wasn't sure how long it would take to recover from surgery. I spent as much time as I could outside. Thankfully, the Bay Area is beautiful and warm in the fall. I was skating in 75-degree weather and soaking up as much sun as possible. Ryan and I would go for rides in his convertible with the top down.

I wasn't about to waste any moment of time on things I didn't love. I also didn't want to marinate in fear.

I recall many women in my triple negative cancer group talking about the time between chemotherapy and surgery. They were all fearful of the cancer coming back once they stopped chemotherapy. I had never even thought about that until I read about it. That entire support group bred a lot of fear. Also, you were not to speak of alternative therapies. It was strictly western medicine. I found it useful for asking questions about navigating certain side effects, sharing beauty tips, and celebrating wins. I finally left the group. I found myself getting immersed in their fears. All of the OMG WHAT IFs were infiltrating my brain. And I, too, began to feel like chemotherapy was my security blanket. What if more cancer grows inside of me or metastasizes to another area of my body while I'm waiting for surgery? Maybe this was a possibility, but deep in my heart I knew I was fine. Rather than live in fear, I just decided to focus on how great I felt. My body was showing me that my tissues were regenerating. My hair was growing! My skin looked better! This was a sign that I had healthy cellular activity. So fuck it. I just decided to focus on being joyful.

The surgery clinic contacted me to go over all of the information that I needed to prepare for surgery—things like when to stop eating and drinking fluids, how to cleanse my skin around the area where incisions would be made, where I would need to check in, and so on. She also spelled out every single step of the procedures I would be having leading up to my 11 a.m. surgery check-in.

I wasn't scared. I was confident in my surgeon's reputation as a total badass. Her confidence in getting this done easily was also comforting. My experience so far was so good, there was nothing to worry about. And honestly, was worrying about future pain the best use of my time? No way! Worrying does not change any outcome. Worrying is a total day-ruiner! My goal was to soak in as much joy as I could and trust that these highly experienced and knowledgeable professionals would do a wonderful job. I believed beyond a shadow of a doubt that this day would go smoothly.

My parents arrived on Saturday the 28th, just two days before my surgery. They had not seen me since my cancer diagnosis. I talked on the phone with my mother every other day, but to date, not face to face. She asked me to do one thing on a regular basis—to let her know I was doing okay. She was very supportive, always listening to the ups and downs of treatment.

Mom was a retired operating room technician, so she understood what went on in and out of the operating room. I also thought that she would know best what kind of post surgical assistance I would need.

I cooked a big meal for my parents. After all, they had spent many hours on the road driving from the southwest border of Washington, all the way to the Bay Area. That entire trip is about 12 hours.

Luckily, we were able to find a lovely Airbnb just two blocks away from where I lived. I was so happy that they could just walk to my house. Everything came together perfectly. It was so comforting to see them both in person, to get my hugs. I had missed them so much and even more throughout this cancer adventure and all the limitations of COVID.

We spent Sunday together just enjoying the day, eating leftover Thanksgiving dinner and resting. Truthfully, we just didn't know what kind of state I would be in after surgery and I wanted to make the most of the time I had with them. I made it a point to end our Sunday night early so that I could put myself to bed early. I had to be up at 6:00 a.m. to shower and get ready for surgery. We had to leave my place no later than 7:15 a.m. to make it to my check-in time at 7:45 a.m.

12

Surgery Day

"From every wound there is a scar, and every scar tells a story. A story that says, "I survived." —Craig Scott

I managed to get a fair amount of sleep the night before and woke up bright and early at 6:00 a.m. I took my shower and cleansed my chest area with Hibiclens, which helps to remove all bacteria from the skin. It felt weird to get up and not drink my tea. I wasn't allowed to have any water.

I would have thrown on a ball gown for this occasion if I had one. Instead, I threw on my sweats and warm things. It was a chilly, but beautiful Northern California fall morning. Comfort felt like the most self-loving thing rather than making a big to-do. "Hey, I'm Cinderfuckinrella, where's the VIP room for lumpectomies? Can you glitter up this left tit for its debut on the surgery table?"

I felt overwhelmed by emotion. Part 2 of 3 in my cancer journey would be over by the end of the day. Who wouldn't be emotional about getting across yet another finish line! With chemo far behind me now, surgery felt like the easiest part of my journey. After all, they'll knock me out and I'll probably wake up with lopsided boobs. I can live with that. This is why sparkles and googly eyes were invented. I seriously didn't know how different my left breast would look from my right. We didn't know exactly how much tissue she would have to remove or how many lymph nodes would be removed.

I wasn't concerned about that part. I just wanted to be alive and done with this portion of my journey.

My parents decided to ride along with us to the hospital. It was about a 20-minute drive from my place to the Carol Ann Read Breast Health Center. The ride started out kind of somber and quiet. I could tell everyone was nervous. I had my concerns, I guess I was just so excited about being closer to the finish line that I wasn't as nervous as I thought I'd be. Reggie was on her way to work that morning, so she met up with us in front of the hospital.

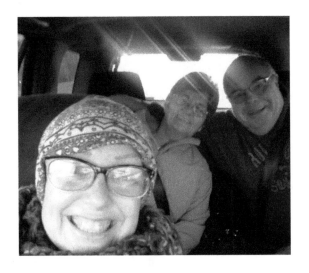

I decided to break up the nervousness and put some dance music on. I kind of fantasized about having a little dance party in the parking garage before I went in, but I knew I'd probably be the only one getting down. I could imagine the confusion of healthcare workers passing by this bald woman dancing around in her sweats. And then I imagined security being called on us for disturbing the peace. Maybe dancing around in a hospital parking garage at 7:30 a.m. with house music bumping and my bald ass busting out some freaky dance moves wouldn't be a good idea. Maybe I should just go in and leave the dancing for later when I actually close this chapter.

We headed from the parking garage to the front of the hospital where Reggie met us. I was feeling kinda special showing up with an entourage! My parents were excited to meet the woman who had hooked me up with my awesome cancer team and took every scary step beside me. They had written her a card and gave her a gift as a token of their appreciation. Their admiration was clear. They had nothing but love and gratitude for Reggie. She had eased their anxiety and shown that I was, indeed, in good hands.

It was time to go inside, so I hugged my parents. I felt both love and nerves. I could almost read Dad's mind—"Goddammit, why does my little girl have to be put through all of this." I knew if they could have taken it all away, they would have. But here we were, and nothing could change that. I just had to accept that there was a reason that was so much bigger than me as to why I was chosen for this cancer.

I turned to Ryan and gave him the biggest hug, letting him know I was going to be all right. "I'm gonna be okay, Squeaks. Just remember, she might run behind schedule so I promise to let you know as much as I can until my phone is taken away from me."

"Okay, Bean. I love you."

And with that we kissed each other and gave each other nose nuzzles. My entourage watched as Reggie and I made our way inside and past the COVID security check.

"How are you feeling? Are you nervous? Excited?!" Reggie asked.

"A little of both, but more excited to cross this off my list. Thanks to you, I know I'm in great hands."

The first part of surgery day was to get something called a wire localization, a procedure that uses a fine wire that almost looks like an acupuncture needle, to mark the exact location of where the original lump was. The technician uses a mammogram to give guidance as to where the clip marker is located to insert the wire. This is done so that the surgeon knows precisely where to make the incision. This makes the surgeon's job much easier and I'm sure less scarring for me.

The whole process took no more than 30 minutes. The nurse assisting at the time was absolutely wonderful. She told me what to expect and that typically there wasn't much pain involved. The technician located the metal clip marking where the original breast tumor was. I was injected with lidocaine in the areas where the wire was to be inserted. The nurse quickly grabbed my hand in an offer of comfort and support during the entire procedure, which was so sweet. But truthfully, I never felt too much except for very slight pinching. It took a few times to get it into the precise location. We were able to see the wire going into my breast and joining up with the metal clip on imaging. Once I was done, I was to be escorted to a shuttle that took me to nuclear medicine to have a radioactive dye injected. The dye travels to the sentinel lymph nodes, which allows my surgeon to identify for biopsy and removal.

The nurse who assisted me, gathered my belongings and wrapped a warm towel around me. I was still in my hospital gown, kinda feeling on display, hoping my wired-up tit ain't falling out. I couldn't have asked for a better nurse; she was so encouraging and told me about her recent cancer journey and how she beat it. She flagged down the shuttle driver and got me completely situated. Before closing the doors, she wished me luck and expressed her confidence that I would do great. The driver had his head out the window and seemed to be having a heated conversation with someone. Once he rolled up the window, he turned to me and said, "Don't they know I'm a shuttle driver, not a therapist!!"

"Good to know. I was planning on telling you my whole life story."

He was quite a character. Do you know where you're going?" he asked.

"Nope!" I said. "I'm new here."

"Okay, I got you. I'll take you there."

I'm so grateful he did because we ended up going through a maze of corridors to get to nuclear medicine. This man knew everyone that he passed by and gave them all shit along the way. I liked this fella.

When we arrived at nuclear medicine, he rang the doorbell. As about a minute rolled by he said, "Where da heck are they?"

He's looking through the window and sees no one.

"Okay, I'll be back. You wait here."

Within five minutes he was back and said, "He's coming for you."

Sure enough, a gentleman opened the door and greeted me. "Hello Ms. Olson, I guess they finished you early! I'll get you another warm blanket and we'll take care of you in just a few minutes."

In the meantime, I took a moment to check in with Ryan to let him know I was done with my wire localization and was now waiting for my injection. I was giving everyone the play-by-play on my Facebook support group as well.

By around 10 a.m. I was finished with my injection. I didn't really feel anything. The nurse who had assisted with the injection escorted me to the pre-surgery waiting area. Again, I'm on display, warm blanket as my shawl, and fancy blue and white hospital gown. That's right, don't hate me because I'm this sexy on a Monday morning after enduring a deep thrust into my breast. Oh, and that scent? Eu de Hibicleans antibacterial soap all over my boobs. Exclusive at Walgreens. My natural pheromones and magnetism have zero bacteria.

There was a bit of a line at the pre-surgery waiting room and the nurse was kind enough to stand in line and alert the office staff of my presence. About 20 minutes later, my registration was complete. However, I was way early. There was a screen on the wall in the waiting area that displayed each surgical room and what surgeon was in each of those rooms. It appeared my surgeon was currently in surgery. When I wasn't called back at the 11 a.m. time, I knew that she was running behind. I alerted Ryan to let him know she was finishing up but I wasn't sure if we would be getting started on time. I let him know I would be shutting my phone off but once I was taken back, that my phone and belongings would be placed in a bag and stashed away.

I turned off my phone and at 11:20 a.m., I was called back to pre-op. One more step closer! I could literally taste the victory! My nurse took me back to a large room with a bed, gave me a new gown and told me to remove my underwear. Come to think of it, I had not had a bowel movement yet. Oh my. I realized that the reason why they had me do this is that people must end up pooping and peeing in the middle of surgery. Please don't let this be me. Great, now I'm nervous about taking a dump in the middle of surgery. Ugh. I hadn't been worked up about this until now!

The nurse ran through all of the pre-op procedures, making sure I took some pain meds and Tylenol. My surgeon popped her head in. I'm so glad I got to see her before we began. My oncologist was supposed to alert her that I was to have my port removed at surgery and somehow that message never made it to my surgeon. My surgeon went over the procedure with me but there was no mention about the port.

"The port is also being removed today right?" I asked.

She said, "Ohhhhhh, I don't have this down for today. Did Dr. G say it was okay?"

"Yes, when she gave me the results for the PET scan, she told me that I could have it taken out and would let you know."

"Is this for reals? Like for really reals?" she asked.

"Yes, I promise. You can contact her if you need to. But she did say it could be removed. I swear."

I damn near began to sweat. I mean, this was the most exciting part of surgery was to get this crazy port out!

"I mean, it's absolutely not a problem to do it! So, let's go ahead and plan it and I'll put a message into her."

Oh, sweet baby Jesus, thank you. Because I've been wanting to break up with this port since the day I got it.

"Besides, we've got to get this thing out. It's been flipping around way too much." My surgeon was also a mind reader!

"Okay, Ellen, your anesthesiologist will be in very soon. Even though we are a little behind schedule, we'll get you in quickly. I'll call Ryan when we are all finished."

"Yay! Thank you!"

This is actually happening! We are doing this! Bye-bye lumps! And good riddance, you annoying port!

The anesthesiologist came in to greet me just minutes later and explained how the anesthesia part worked and that I would have a tube inserted in my throat for breathing.

"You won't know that it's there, but you might notice in the next day or so that your throat might get mildly sore. Some people don't notice at all, but just wanted to give you a heads-up that it can happen. Just in case you do experience nausea from the anesthesia, we are going to give you some Zofran to keep you from feeling sick tonight. You may want to take a laxative later."

Since me and Zofran know each other really well now, I was armed with MiraLAX. Just you try and come at me, brick turds!

When the surgery room was ready, my anesthesiologist wheeled me back. As we entered into a dark hallway filled with UV lights, the room temperature went from wonderfully tropical to freezing. I tried not to think about how this reminded me of past horror films of people being disemboweled, but my head kind of went there.

As I was wheeled into the surgical room, I was greeted by a couple of people who would be attending in surgery. Everyone introduced themselves and chatted with me as they continued with preparations.

One of the attending nurses pulled out her phone and said, "Okay Ellen, what are we going to listen to during your surgery?"

"Oh, is that Spotify?"

"Yes ma'am!"

"Okay, can we do Tribe Called Quest? Low End Theory?"

My anesthesiologist gave his seal of approval with an "Awwww yeah!"

I heard another voice in the background, "Yes! Let's do it!"

"If you guys don't like it, then Deee-Lite would be fun too!"

"Oh yeah, Deee Lite!"

I guess whatever lovely drugs my anesthesiologist had just injected made me a bit chatty and I started talking about my Spotify playlist for roller skating. Then skating became the topic as the surgery team continued preparation.

At some point, I drifted off into sleep and when I awoke, I was greeted by someone who asked me a few questions about pain and when I answered coherently, "no pain." I was moved to another area and greeted by a young man who loved to chat it up as much as I do. PERFECT!

He wheeled from side to side on his chair as he multitasked. Are you feeling any pain Ms. Olson?" he asked.

"No, I actually feel good. Just a bit tired."

"Perfect, the feeling tired is normal and you may continue to feel a bit groggy. I have some great news for you. Doctor says you have no cancer in your lymph nodes."

Wait. What? You mean those giant lumps that once looked like an alien trying to escape out of my armpit in the form of cancer are gone?

I'm not gonna lie, I did a happy dance right there in my recovery bed. Improvised, of course, because I could not get my left arm up and shimmying was not an option. I looked more like a disabled, one-winged bird trying to take flight from its ass. Makes no difference. Attitude sells. And that excitement I threw into that dance made it pure perfection.

"Once your doctor gets the pathology report, they will go over all of the details for you."

Oh, that's right. I have to wait a week or so to get the results. I'll have no idea if I had actually achieved a complete pathological response to chemotherapy. I have no idea if there was any cancer left in my breast.

Of course, you have to run through a series of things in order to be released. I think the important thing was being able to walk to the bathroom on my own and report that I was able to urinate. Check! I did that without any assistance! I also wasn't going to be released if I seemed inebriated or if my vitals didn't check out good. So far, I was making total sense, could hold conversations, and vitals looked good. I was informed that my surgeon had contacted Ryan, so he and my parents knew that I was doing okay.

One of Reggie's old coworkers showed up to check up on me. That woman had an army of people she could call to do a face-to-face check-in and report back to her. Luckily, I was up and in good spirits and close to being released.

Being amidst a pandemic can feel somewhat lonely because you can't have your loved ones by your side. So, for me, to have an actual visitor brought me a lot of joy. I know it was her intention to make sure I was okay, but those check-ins did more for me than she knew.

I have no idea how much time passed by in post-op. But between visiting with staff and getting through my release checklist, the time seemed to fly by. Before I knew it, a lovely woman appeared with a wheelchair to roll me out to the pick-up area and unite me with my loved ones.

I'm sure that for the first time, Ryan and my family found my chattiness very comforting. I wasn't face-down drooling or in pain. I was alive, happy and celebrating a big win. Two out of three down.

That night, I got home and finally had a bowel movement. I looked down and staring back at me was the bluest turd I have ever seen in my life. I just shit a Smurf-blue radioactive turd. Never in my life did I think I would want to check that off of my bucket list, but I can now report that this is an achievement that many cannot say they accomplished in their lifetime. Suddenly, I feel special. I couldn't wait to report to Reggie!

Mom and I took a moment to check out the incisions near my left armpit and my left breast. We were completely astonished by the lack of swelling. While the areas that were incised had some bruising, it didn't look scary at all. Ryan was impressed. My left breast looked untouched. Nothing about it looked like any tissue was removed. No divots, no dimples. It would be interesting over the next few weeks to see how everything looked once I healed.

Strangely enough, the area where my port used to sit felt empty in a strange way. It had occupied space on the right side of my cleavage for six months. It felt like a giant growth had been removed. I was relieved that I would no longer need to deal with inconvenience and pain of the port flipping. Removing the port was like a sign that my cancer was gone and would never return.

All things considered; I got a good night's sleep. I never had to take any pain meds except for some ibuprofen.

The next day, my parents checked in to see how I was doing, and I asked them to come over so that we could go for a walk.

A few days prior to surgery, my naturopath had me start a regimen of arnica and staphysagria pellets, which aid in wound healing and decrease swelling and bruising. I took these pellets three days prior to surgery and daily until the bruising went away. I witnessed the power of these pellets literally overnight. Because when I woke up the day after, the bruising and swelling had decreased by about 60 percent. No exaggeration.

My parents arrived, astonished by my energy and how great I looked. I had to show my mom the overnight difference in my bruising and swelling. She couldn't believe the difference.

I felt well enough to get out for a two-mile walk the day after surgery. My parents joined me to make sure I was steady on my feet. On the days after surgery, we went for walks together, sometimes up to three miles. I only did what felt right, never pushed and just wanted to soak up as much sun as possible.

I did have a couple of days where I felt exhausted and didn't do much. Those days, my parents never left my side. Being the empath that I am, I felt their emotions. How unfair it was that their daughter had to go through cancer! The fear of the possibility that something could go horribly wrong. This was the first time that they had seen me through my journey. And although they witnessed my strength and courage, there were times when they could see how stretched I was physically, emotionally, and financially. But underneath it all, my spirit was alive and well and I'm sure it gave them comfort knowing that I would never back down, that I would win this cancer in a staring contest.

My parents stayed with me for a week after surgery. I thought maybe I would need more help. I didn't know. Planning for the worst was good. We didn't need it and instead used that time to order in meals, watch movies together, and catch up on storytelling. It was something I really missed living far away.

When it was time for them to go, I cried. But luckily, Ryan and I made plans to drive up to see them for the holidays. And in addition, I would get to see my brothers, my sister-in-law and niece. It meant everything to me to spend a quiet holiday with them and to have a nice break. The timing of my surgery healing couldn't have been better.

Exactly two weeks after my surgery, I met with my oncologist to go over pathology reports and to see how my blood counts were doing. My blood counts looked like they were steadily rising and I was feeling really good. In fact, the scarring was looking to be very minimal.

I had prepared myself to hear good news since my post-surgery paperwork stated that my lymph nodes had no cancer. Well, that wasn't completely true.

My oncologist reported to me that I had a really wonderful response to chemotherapy. My breast tissue, the OG tumor showed no cancer activity in the pathology reports. However, two of the eight of my sentinel lymph nodes tested showed a small cluster of cancer cells. The first one showed .8 mm of micrometastasis and the second showed .2 mm of micrometastasis. This means that I didn't have a complete pathological response to chemotherapy, but three lymph nodes were removed during surgery, taking out the ones that had the cancer. This should all be good, right? Well, yes and no. Yes because they *think* all of the cancer is gone BUT those lymph nodes in my chest wall—the ones near my trachea? Those couldn't be biopsied. Nobody can say for sure if those lymph nodes had cleared since two of the sentinel nodes did not clear. At that time, she didn't feel that I would need any additional chemotherapy, thank goodness. But she thought that immunotherapy would be a great insurance policy to make sure every single cancer cell was accounted for.

While I was so grateful that she wanted to make sure that she did everything in her power to make sure I wouldn't have a recurrence and stay cancer free, I will admit I was totally sad to find out that there was some cancer left and that further treatment would be advised to ensure my survival.

The radiation I would receive once I returned from the holidays would kill off any cancer, but there was more concern of rogue cells splitting off and metastasizing elsewhere.

I was told that if I was approved for immunotherapy, that I would be getting infusions every three weeks for anywhere from six months to possibly two years. My heart sank. Now you are saying that once I finish radiation I'll still need to be on treatments. I thought I was going to be done. What the fuck cancer. I thought we had an agreement. I did EVERYTHING that I could do to get rid of you. How could even the smallest amount have survived?

My oncologist said she would talk with the tumor board for suggestions and also put me in touch with an oncologist from UCSF for a second opinion. Before I begin radiation in January, I would have more concrete answers.

While I knew that deep down, I responded so well to treatment given all that had to be dealt with, the idea of doing more treatment was devastating. I cried all the way out to the car and called Ryan. "Okay, well, just keep remembering, we're in a way better place than you were and that you have options." Ryan was always good about pointing out the number of options I had. If one door closed, there were hundreds of other doors wide open. And he was right.

I also spoke to my dad. I could hear his optimism, but I could also hear his disappointment. He wanted me to be finished with treatments just as badly as I wanted. If he could have kicked the shit out of that cancer for me, he would have. I knew in his mind he was having words with it. "You piece of shit, no good low life cancer. Get away from my daughter." It was like a nightmare, stalker boyfriend. Only sadly, he couldn't chase it down with a baseball bat or call the police. I had to do it myself.

Over the next few weeks, I decided to take a break from it all. I would wait to see what the panel of doctors would come up with and I would do my own research about things I could do to keep it away. I took the time to heal after surgery, went on walks, hikes and skated as often as I could. I even started running again. Movement brought me joy.

The time that I got to spend with my family during the holidays meant so much to me. It was the first time I REALLY felt relaxed. I slept in. I went on a couple of runs with my brother. We had, what I considered, the best Christmas in years. In fact, we had such a lovely time, we decided to stay an extra day.

After I returned home, I had a video meeting with an oncologist from UCSF who gave me a second opinion. She informed me that I was actually stage 4 and that because I was stage 4 I would not be able to qualify for immunotherapy. Her recommendation was to put me on a chemotherapy pill for six months and that maybe I would qualify for another immunotherapy trial.

When I informed her that I was quite active and ate an extremely healthy diet along with all of the other holistic approaches I took, she informed me that these things would greatly increase my chances of survival.

Chances of survival? I really hate that doctors have to bring up the possibility that I may die. Guess what, we are all going to die. But when you plant the death seed in someone's brain during cancer, they have doubts and begin to lose hope.

I then met with my oncologist and we discussed my meeting with the second-opinion oncologist. I asked her about the stage 4 diagnosis.

"It's a bit of a grey area for some doctors. I treated you as a stage 3 patient and you responded very well. I want to ensure your success going forward and will use everything we've got to drastically reduce your risk in recurrence. The Xeloda pill will be good for you and is typically well tolerated. There are some side effects. You can experience nausea, diarrhea, fatigue and it can affect your blood counts. People tend to have issues with hands and feet drying out, peeling and cracking. So you'll need to stay hydrated and keep creams on your hands and feet as often as possible."

I didn't like the sounds of any of this. More chemo. It sounded like I would have some of the same effects as regular chemotherapy but just not as intense.

"We would like to have you get started about three weeks after you are finished with radiation."

I took it all in and decided from there that I would do a ton of research on other treatments that wouldn't further deteriorate my body. I would take my time to do this through my radiation treatments. Nothing about more chemo felt right to me.

13

Laser Beams of Love— Adventures in Radiation

After meeting with my radiation oncologist, from what I understood, at most I would feel tired towards the end. My skin might become sensitive and possibly burn. Because they would be radiating near my trachea, my throat could get a bit sore and inflamed. It was also possible that I would develop a little bit of a cough towards the end. Okay, this sounds like a cakewalk next to chemotherapy.

The plan was to go every morning for 7 a.m. appointments Monday through Friday. That way, I'd have the rest of the day to myself. I would start my radiation treatments on January 11th and end on February 23rd. Just six weeks. The appointments would take no more than 20 minutes. I can do this.

Prior to beginning radiation, I had to come in for a walk-through and to get tiny dot tattoos. This would help the radiation technicians get me lined up on the table for my radiation treatments. I also had to hold my breath so that the radiation would miss my heart. Scary sounding, but these professionals had it down to an exact science.

My first day of radiation was as easy as described. Once they lined me up on the table, they left the room, instructed me to hold my breath and the machine would circle around me. It would do three passes. During each of my radiation treatments, I would recite over and over in my head: "These are my laser beams of love, burning out all that no longer serves me." My good friend Catherine had told me what she recited when she received radiation. And I decided to use her idea. I loved the idea of having laser beams of love burning out the old, useless bullshit.

Each day, I would wake up at 5:45 a.m. and remove all of the creams and oils I had applied the night before from my left breast, underarm, and in between both breasts. I would take my supplements, put on my workout clothes and head into radiation. I always wanted to jazz myself up before going, so I'd blast some of my favorite old-school hip hop or house music all the way to the cancer center.

When I left my house at 6:25 a.m., it was dark out. I appreciated that people left their Christmas lights up well into February so I could enjoy the sparkles along the way to my radiation appointments.

I would arrive at 6:45 a.m., get changed into a gown, and just around 7 a.m. one of my radiation techs fetched me for treatment. It would take no longer than five minutes for them to line me up perfectly and, once they were ready, they would leave the room and begin treatment. Over the loudspeaker, they would instruct me when to hold my breath. At first, I wasn't any good at it. I hadn't been in the practice of holding my breath for any length of time. But as each day passed, I got really good at it. Maybe I was just nervous in the beginning, but holding my breath was never an issue after the first week.

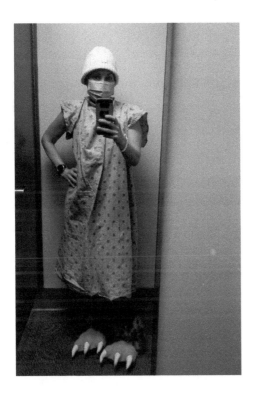

By 7:15 a.m., I was finished, and I would return to the changing area to put my steroid and calendula cream mixture all over the areas where I was radiated, put my clothes on and leave. By the time I walked outside, it was daylight.

After I was finished, I would head out to my workouts. Sometimes I'd go for a run or long walk at the beach. I'd do online strength-training classes or dance classes. And many times, I'd hit the basketball court for some roller skating. It thrilled me to get all my exercising out of the way because, typically, I'd have more appointments to go to throughout the day. At that time, I wanted to support my body as much as possible. I was getting acupuncture, chiropractic adjustments and massage, physical therapy, AND I was still doing follow-up appointments with my radiation oncologist, naturopath, therapist, and oncologist. I felt like a full-time patient. At times I'd have three appointments a day.

About three weeks into radiation, I started getting a sore throat. The best way I could describe the pain at first was very similar to strep throat. Not fun, but I managed okay for the first week and a half. The fatigue began to kick in by my fourth week of radiation. Each day, my throat got worse, to the point that it would throb uncontrollably in pain. I had come back from radiation one day in so much pain, unable to eat solid foods, and even drinking juices felt like I was pouring alcohol onto a bad wound. I needed relief. I had leftover pain meds from surgery that I hadn't even touched. I called my nurse navigator asking for suggestions. She told me to take the ibuprofen and Norco that I had left over from surgery. It worked a little bit each day, it gradually got worse, and those pain meds gave me zero relief.

At week four, I had bloodwork done and my throat was examined. Everything looked good at that moment; there was no sign of infection and my blood counts held strong. I was given a prescription for something called magic mouthwash, which contained viscous lidocaine and Benadryl. I would drink this before drinking water to ease the difficulty of swallowing from the pain. After a few days, the magic mouthwash stopped working. About a week and a half before I would finish radiation, the pain became so intense. One morning, I showed up to my appointment in tears. The pain was intense, and the throbbing was out of control. At that point, swallowing water was difficult and I could barely get fluids down. I had to get through this radiation appointment. If I skipped it, I would have to push out an extra day. I was going to finish this on the 23rd of February. How the heck was I going to be able to hold my breath? My technicians offered to give me a moment to collect myself. I gave the thumbs-up that I was ready.

"Okay, take a breath in."

I took that breath in and held my breath. As the machine slowly moved over my head, tears streamed down my face. I can do this. I can hold my breath and we won't have to stop. These are my laser beams of love, burning out all of the negative shit in my life. And obviously, they did their job because it felt like someone had poured gasoline down my throat and lit it on fire.

When I was finished, I spoke to the staff and asked if they had any other tools in their toolbelt to get me some relief from the pain.At that point, I was given a prescription for oxycodone. While it didn't do much to relieve the pain, it did make me sleep a lot. And I guess I would rather sleep through the pain, then actually feel it all day.

Each day it got worse. The pain was relentless. And on top of it all, I began to have GI issues. I was taking laxatives because the oxy was constipating. My stomach started to sound consistently like there were cats screaming inside and I ended up having diarrhea all day. I felt like maybe it was an infection. At the same time, I began having difficulty urinating. I got to a point where I was unable to swallow fluids.

When I had reached the point of being unable to hydrate myself, I had to start receiving IV fluids right after my radiation treatments. I would bring meal replacement shakes so that I could get calories in, and sometimes, organic mint ice cream was the only thing that I could get down. I found the cold, creamy mint to be soothing.

About seven days before I was to finish my radiation, I was given morphine with my IV fluids. The nurse who was administering the medication told me that I would feel better within minutes of receiving the morphine. An hour after he administered the morphine, I asked when I would start to feel relief. He said, "You should have felt it already. You don't feel anything?"

"No."

Ugh. I felt totally jipped. Not only did it not give relief, but I also didn't even get high. At least if I was going to be in pain, I'd rather have been so out of my head that I didn't even notice the pain.

I was prescribed viscous lidocaine and, thankfully, as I was receiving my fluids, the pharmacist delivered it to me. I was to take the viscous lidocaine right before I drank my shakes or water. It sort of helped but gave me a window of about five minutes to get it all down. It was not enough time for someone who had difficulty swallowing, but enough to get something down.

On a Saturday morning, the weekend right before I was to finish up my last two radiation treatments, I woke up with a 101.7-degree fever. I felt like someone ran me over and then backed over me twice. Is this COVID? I hope not. I took a Tylenol to bring down the fever. I felt like I might possibly have a stomach and urinary tract infection. Maybe my throat was infected and possibly the reason why I was in so much pain. Whatever it was, it wasn't good. I was worried about having a systemic infection.

I called the after-hours line at the cancer center and spoke to the on-call physician. She thought possibly it was an infection but wanted me to check in later if the fever came back. Truthfully, the Tylenol did make me feel a bit better and seemed to relieve the throat pain just a little bit. Once the Tylenol wore off, the fever came back, and this time it felt like my throat was closing up. I called the on-call physician back and she decided to prescribe me a strong six-day antibiotic.

Poor Ryan had been going back and forth with me all week trying to help. On top of it, his job had become increasingly stressful with workloads doubling. He couldn't get a break. I told him to stay home, that I would assemble a team to help me out.

My good friend Nancy offered to come check on me and picked up my antibiotic. I took two as instructed, along with another Tylenol. Almost immediately, I felt a difference. By Sunday evening, my throat was feeling better.

Monday arrived and I had only two radiation sessions left. But because I had reported having a fever over the weekend, the cancer center had to take huge precautions to keep me away from other patients while awaiting my COVID test results. I had to get my

COVID test at the drive-up facility at Sutter Health and then head over to the cancer center to get fluids and radiation. I had to contact one of the staff members to escort me past the COVID check and take me to my private room to be given IV fluids. Although my throat was still hurting, I decided to stop taking all pain meds because I felt like I was taking so many things at once. I felt like my body was on toxic overload and just needed to do its job. So many medicines interact with organ function and I wanted my body to heal as it naturally knows how to do.

Once I was done with receiving fluids, I was escorted through another entrance away from patients to receive radiation.

Eyes on the prize. I'm about to cross this finish line. Once I get through today. Tomorrow will be my last.

Once I finished my session, I was escorted out the back entrance where Ryan picked me up. It felt like a long day and all I wanted to do was rest. I drank the rest of my liquids, put myself to bed early and got a good night's sleep.

Since I had gone completely off all pain meds and laxatives, the only thing I was taking was my antibiotics. I felt tired, but well enough to drive myself to radiation. My COVID test had arrived and it was negative. My technician called from the cancer center to have me come in for my last appointment about an hour earlier. My last day. This is the last day of the brutal race that I had been running for nine fucking months.

Thankfully, I could drink fluids and even got a smoothie down that day. I know my body and I truly believe that I had a throat infection that traveled from my throat, through my GI tract, down to my urinary tract because by my third day of antibiotics, I could pee again and my stomach stopped making angry, growling cat noises.

I also felt less brain fog. All of those meds were messing with me. Our bodies want to heal themselves; we just have to support ourselves in the best way possible and trust that it can do the job. I knew, despite everything I had been through over the last nine months, that I had given my body the support that it needed in order to heal.

The entire gang at the radiation clinic greeted me in celebration of my last day of radiation. I received a certificate of completion signed by everyone there. My last treatment was somewhat bittersweet. The technicians were phenomenal and always paid attention to my comfort. I have to say the staff was so wonderfully compassionate and extremely helpful during the worst of my days.

Even though radiation wasn't as lengthy as chemo, it was by far the most challenging for me. I did feel poisoned by it. I was heavily fatigued during the last three weeks. I ended up with an infection. My esophagus had suffered burns. The skin on my collarbone also suffered intense burns, even with my extreme diligence of applying my healing creams two to four times a day.

In the midst of my radiation treatments, my naturopathic oncologist ordered some blood tests. My iodine, Vitamin D, selenium, ferritin, High Sensitivity C-reactive protein Galectin-3, and a three-month overall glucose reading. She also ordered a Biocept test, which would detect any circulating tumor cells in my bloodstream. Biocept tests are crucial in monitoring anyone who has cancer or has finished cancer treatments. It can help with early detection of recurrence or metastasis.

Because I was receiving radiation during the bloodwork, I wasn't expecting superb results. During that time, I had just started to feel normal after chemotherapy and my aches and pains had diminished. BUT radiation increases inflammation, so I imagine the combination of coming off of chemo and doing radiation would show some type of inflammation in my body. No high hopes here.

Around the first week of February, I received the results of my blood work. I was a little nervous, but better to know than to bury my head in the sand.

My naturopathic oncologist began our meeting by asking me, "Okay, Ellen, where do you want me to start?"

"Go with what you have ready first!" I said.

"Ellen, your Biocept test came back clear with zero circulating tumor cells!"

Holy fucking shit. Am I dreaming? Did she just say zero? I had her repeat it again and she confirmed again, I was clear.

"Zero? Oh my God!!! Wow! I'm so happy!!!" She didn't know it but I was crying tears of joy.

"Next up, all of your inflammatory markers were in normal, healthy ranges!" She had explained the differences in my bloodwork from when I received my first tests back in July and the gigantic differences during radiation. My iron still needed to increase a little bit and because it was winter, my Vitamin D was slightly low. My white blood counts still needed to recover from chemotherapy. The fact that my inflammatory markers went down was nothing short of fanfuckingtastic!

This meant I would have a fighting chance at not getting cancer again as long as these numbers stayed in normal, healthy ranges. Cancer can't breed when the immune system is healthy and when there is no inflammation present. It needs a nasty environment to survive.

The fact that these blood tests came back so healthy barely two months after surgery and three months after chemotherapy was incredible news. If I could get healthy DURING aggressive cancer treatments, then I can only imagine how much healthier I could be without being on treatments.

Those numbers really showed me how all of my hard work had paid off. So I decided to decline the chemotherapy pill to focus on healing. I wanted to improve my blood counts and get this body strong enough to fight anything. All of my hard work during treatment is an example of how the human body responds. If you treat it with respect, eat well, exercise, and integrate a healthy mindfulness practice, you can fight off any disease. If you do the opposite, the body responds with pain, chronic illness, fatigue, and disease.

Now that I had all the tools in place, I knew that my body had the ability to heal itself. After all that I had endured, I felt the highest act of self-love was to trust in my body to heal and use its own ability to fight off illness.

When I began telling my family and friends that I wouldn't be taking the chemo pill, I felt relieved and free. No more feeling like shit. No more fighting to get my white blood counts to go up. No more fatigue. I get to live my life and I can get my strength back again.

For days after, I cried. This means I'm done. I fucking did it. I beat cancer like a total badass.

14

I Had Cancer—
It Never Had Me

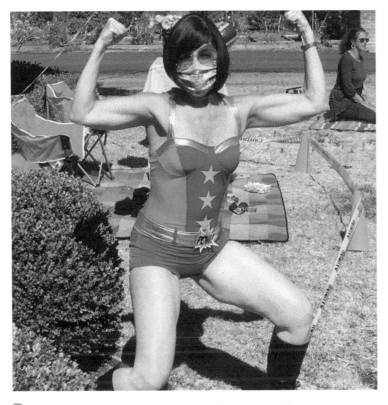

R̲ight after radiation, I continued to see Emil, my acupuncturist, and my chiropractor to continue the healing process

and to give my body support as I began boosting my workouts.

One day, I showed up to my chiropractic appointment and my chiropractor asked me to pick a card from her tarot deck. We're both very intuitive, super spiritual sisters who love holistic healing. It was no accident that the universe matched her to be my chiropractor. We speak the same language when it comes to health and spirituality.

Once she was finished doing her magical adjustment on me, I headed to the deck to pick my card. I shifted the cards around, shuffling and asking for the right card to show up. As I fanned the cards out, one card literally jumped out at me. The card read: "Your heart has a heightened connection with the higher realms of consciousness and light. A blessing, empowerment and positive omen shall enter your world. Doors will open for you. Abundance and prosperity are headed your way. Take care of your heart. Ask for spiritual assistance, and it shall be granted. Something negative is going to transform into something very positive."

I sat there, staring at the card, taking a deep breath, knowing with certainty what the card meant.

My breast cancer diagnosis is the negative thing that is transforming into something positive. It has since the very beginning. Doors have opened for me from the beginning of and throughout my treatment and continue to do so. My heart is open. I continued to meet people who offered to help me in my healing journey.

My cancer journey had really sucky moments, but I chose to take the lessons I needed to learn from it. I always believe when something bad happens, no matter how awful it may be, that we get to learn and grow from those awful experiences. It gives us the opportunity to come out shining. I fucking made it through nine months of torturous treatments and, instead of feeling victimized, I never once let it get me down. I set my goals and believed I would come out of my cancer treatments knowing that if I could beat cancer, I could do anything. I want to help others get through their journey and come out the other side renewed.

In many ways, I'm grateful for the lessons cancer taught me. The experience wised me up and I'm a better human for it. I spent a lot of time eliminating all emotional and physical toxins in my life that were weighing me down. I continue to remind myself that it's okay to not be perfect or to try to make everyone happy. I need to be happy first.

I never once backed down. I came out stronger. Each day that passes, I feel better than the day before. Sometimes I feel as if I had never gone through nine months of brutal, deteriorating treatments. I look at it with this perspective: The forest of bad thoughts, emotions, beliefs and behaviors within me was burned and a bunch of new trees were planted. And I refuse to dump more deteriorating chemicals into my body so I can continue watering those beautiful, new, planted trees.

Beating cancer doesn't mean you are off the hook. Many cancers have a risk for recurrence or showing up elsewhere in the body. I am in for a lifetime of prevention. And I will continue to research and educate myself on all of the ways I can keep my body resilient to cancer and illness. I want to share what I've learned with others so that they can win and keep on winning just as I did.

I realized through this whole journey that we, as a society, are not set up to be successful at living balanced, healthy lives. This is why we get sick. We work long hours. We have little time for ourselves and for our friends and families. By the time we get home at night, we barely have time to cook a healthy meal. And there are really no healthy fast-food options available. We barely have time to exercise or think of nutrition. And even if we did have time, we're too tired and stressed. This is not okay. Yet we believe it's okay because this is the way it has always been. That is utter bullshit. We need more time for our health, for our families, and to enjoy life. We weren't gifted this opportunity of living on this earth to throw it away on stressful commutes and jobs.

If we want to avoid chronic illness or cancer, we must take inventory of our daily lives, the people we surround ourselves with, and our wellness practices. This means having a mindfulness practice, finding ways to reduce the stress, making time for yourself so that you can be of service to others, have a regular exercise regimen, eat organic meals, reduce your radiation exposure, use biohacking equipment like a PEMF mat and plug in radiation protection devices that help reduce radiation exposure in your home. Reduce all the chemicals in your home. Use organic, toxin-free skin care, grooming, and cleaning products in your home. Get in the practice of putting yourself to bed at night so that you can get eight hours of sleep. Turn off your screens and slow down 30 minutes to an hour before bedtime. Stop medicating yourself with drugs and alcohol. Build a life you don't need to escape from. Allow yourself to feel your emotions and cry. Get it out. Scream into a pillow. Get those emotions out of your body. Don't avoid your emotions as that shit will manifest as illness.

Telling someone not to cry is like telling someone to hold their poop in. You have to get it all out of your body! Cry it out, scream it out! Throw rocks! This is one of the most wonderful ways you can heal.

I used to be really good at holding in my emotions, I never felt safe expressing them. I know my cancer manifested in my body because of stress. Stress can be equally as dangerous as smoking cigarettes, eating a poor diet, and not exercising.

From the words of someone who stared death in the face, my advice is to get out and live life. Call on the ones you love and tell them why you love them. Share one of your favorite memories with them. Do something out of your comfort zone. Get comfortable with loving yourself inside and out. Stop giving other people power over you. This means being a pushover, choosing to do something out of guilt, or hanging onto anger over someone who doesn't deserve to take up space in your heart. Be okay with fucking up and owning your fuck ups. Because when you can admit to someone that you messed up and are willing to change your behavior or solve the problem, both people can heal. I've experienced how healing it is to admit my mistakes and my willingness to correct them. I feel good and the other person feels heard. Drop that ego and remember that love and kindness always wins.

I know my cancer came to me from years of self-sabotage, being a pushover, taking care of others before myself, being hard on myself, not seeing the beauty that was staring back at me in the mirror. I worked out too hard and put my body in agony because I didn't like the way I looked. I didn't feel like I was ever doing enough and that I could do better. Sure, I ate right, and I exercised, but my poor soul was just too tired.

This cancer diagnosis woke me up and taught me so much about how to live my life better, how to accept and love myself even more.

I had cancer. It never had me. This may sound crazy, but I believe it was a blessing in disguise. A gift of a new life. And I just can't be mad about that.

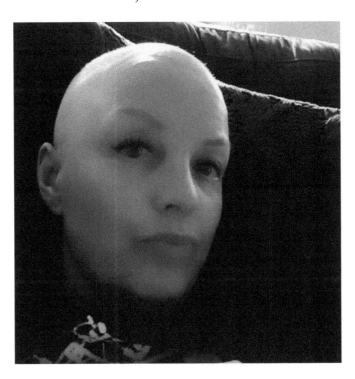

15

Ellen's Checklist for Successfully and Joyfully Surviving Cancer

To my dearest cancer thrivers! I want to share my checklist for assembling and getting the help you need. I feel that we need to all walk into our appointments confident that we have all the support we need so that we can ease ourselves into the journey.

This is my checklist. Use whatever you wish. There is no one right way to walk through cancer. This is YOUR journey, and you must do what feels best for you. Also, understand that doing the exact same thing I did may not produce the same outcome. Know that your results may vary. Every person's genetic makeup is unique. I started this journey with a strong body; you may too. Or you may begin from a different place.

The biggest thing you can possess in this journey is your will to live and relentless tenacity. Never back down!

You can decide to do what you want to do. It's your body and your choice. If you truly want to go 100% holistic, know that your support group and your oncologist may disagree. If your oncologist does disagree, find another. There are amazing doctors out there who will respect your wishes to do what feels best for you. This is YOUR life!

Always remember that YOU are not a statistic. You don't have to discuss mortality rates. And you can ask your team not to give you a death sentence. I think this is rude and unfair to anyone dealing with cancer.

I found that cancer really gave me perspective on what I really wanted out of life. What I realized is that I wasn't happy with certain aspects, like I didn't like my job.

Instead of seeing cancer as a death sentence, can you see it as a life sentence? After all, you are still alive!! What excites you? Is there something you've been saying for years that you'd like to do but you haven't done it? Do you want to change jobs or take up painting? Learn a language? While your cancer treatments might slow you down, look at this slow time as an opportunity to connect with what lights you up. Do you have any goals that you want to set?

For instance, I wanted to study to become a fitness instructor and learn some Spanish during the days I was stuck on the couch. I wanted to learn how to draw better, so one of my friends sent me a book called *How to Draw Cool Stuff.* Maybe you would like to paint or visit nature more often. Think of ways that you can create your own little oasis amidst your cancer treatments. Write down a list of goals. Maybe you want to completely rearrange your life! That's perfectly okay too! Listen to what your heart desires and write it down. Since the cancer journey forces us to be brave, this means you can be brave for any adventure you want!

I wrote an entire business plan and began tackling it one by one. I designed my skin care website and began studying for my fitness exam! I was also writing notes for this book!

Sometimes people feel better having a purpose and others want to simplify their lives. Whatever feels good to you, take time to write about it and design your plan throughout your journey. Have an exciting goal waiting for when you finish your cancer treatments. Keep your focus and your eyes on the prize! Journal about your goals during treatments. Keep writing and stay excited!

Important Questions To ask Yourself As You Begin Your Cancer Journey

Upon diagnosis, make a list of everything you will need help with.

- Do you need rides? Do you need someone to take care of your children?

- Will you need assistance with meals? Can you take a leave from work?
- Is your job so stressful that you definitely do not need it hovering over your head like a black cloud during cancer treatments?
- Do you need supplements or access to other medication that you can't afford?
- Can you meet basic expenses during your cancer journey?
- Would you like to appoint someone to alert your loved ones of your diagnosis and assemble help?

Take a moment to list all of the things that you would like help with during your journey.

I know that asking for help is really tough. I am not a person who easily accepted help. I worried about asking for too much or burdening others. Know that you are worthy of receiving love and assistance. We are not in this world alone for a reason! You will be amazed at how others will show up for you and how much they do want to help. THIS is how you assemble your cartel of love!

Here is my list that I wrote out for my necessities:

1. Set up a Facebook support group. Use a photo of yourself and communicate what the support group is used for: Thank you everyone for being

a part of the cheer squad! I am overwhelmed by your love and generosity! This support group is a place to organize assistance for me during my journey. I ask that you NOT call or text me and instead use this space to ask questions and post your supportive words. I need to reserve my phone use for doctors and communicating with those who are organizing assistance.

Please respect these wishes:

- Please contact me here first before connecting me with health practitioners and/or other cancer survivors.
- Please DO not offer unsolicited medical and supplemental advice unless you have experience in oncology or have successfully survived my type of cancer.
- Please understand that it may take time for me to return messages or that I may not acknowledge your message. This does not mean I haven't read it; it means I'm overwhelmed and must focus on my self care. Know that your loving messages are seen and very much appreciated!
- Be respectful of my choices. Challenging my cancer journey is not appreciated.
- Thank you for joining me in kicking cancer's ass!

2. Enlist helpers to do these things:

- Set up a meal train—a group of people who can bring you food when you are unable to cook.

- Set up a GoFundMe platform to help with out-of-pocket expenses and meeting basic cost-of-living expenses.

- Get someone to research your health practitioners. Make sure they are reputable and, IF you plan to integrate holistic therapies, that your doctors respect your wish to support yourself holistically through conventional treatments.

- Get three to five of your favorite people to help assemble your team of helpers. For example: Have one person set up a ride schedule, one person to organize child care, one person to organize people to run errands for you and/or tidy up your home.

- Set up a list of things you will need throughout your journey. You may lose your hair so caps and wigs can be fun. You can ask for supplements that can be costly when added up. Make a thorough list with links and post to your Facebook group. You can also enlist someone to find links for these items for you.

- If you need supplemental income, look into (or have someone look into) state disability programs, Social Security, and paid family medical leave. Your spouse/partner may also be able to take time off and receive funds as your caretaker.
- Get your will, advanced directives, and power of attorney in place. I know this sounds awful and morbid but, no matter what, we all need this done. You may at times not be able to make decisions for yourself and will need to appoint someone that you trust to make decisions.
- If you go this route, find your holistic team. Research naturopaths who are well versed in oncology. There are many places who can work with you online.

You will not read anything good about your cancer. There is a lot of fear-based information out there. Instead, you can find inspiration in these books: *Radical Remission* by Kelly A. Turner, *How to Starve Cancer Without Starving Yourself* by Jane McClelland, and *The Metabolic Approach to Cancer* by Dr. Nasha Winters. You will find much relief in knowing there are many survivors out there who beat the worst odds and came out healthy. Feed your mind with these pieces of inspiration!"

3. **Set yourself up to feel like a badass every day!**
   What are the songs that make your hair stand on your arms, the songs that make you want to dance? You need something inspiring, music that makes you want to get out of bed. Make yourself a badass playlist.

   This is the soundtrack that will get you out of bed every day. The thing that will get you jazzed about living. Music can help turn a bad mood into a better one with just one song. Get that playlist together and play it as often as you can.

4. **Set some daily intentions and read them out loud every day as often as you can.**
   You've got to plant the seed in your head that you are amazing and kicking ass even when it doesn't feel that way. Here's an example of mine: I am a powerful healing machine and I feel good! I am strong, I'm unstoppable and I'm healthy!! Today, I'll get out for a walk and balance with rest! I am grateful to be alive! I am loved and I can do anything I set my mind to!"

   When we plant seeds like this, it can really raise our vibration. So instead of being tired and feeling low, when you put on your playlist and you read this out loud, that badass is going to start coming out.

You also don't have to be a rockstar every day. You can say something like, "I'm a powerful healer who will spend the day enjoying movie time on the couch and relaxing in my pajamas! I deserve this time to rejuvenate and rest! You can be just as excited about lying under the covers doing absolutely nothing.

5. **Get moving!**
It can be really difficult to move around especially after receiving chemo. I would wake up each day and set a fitness goal. Even if it was to get up every couple of hours and walk up and down the block. I researched online dance classes and workout classes. I didn't set high expectations—the goal is to move. So put that playlist on and dance like no one is watching! Make a goal to get some movement in every day if you can. If you absolutely can't then that's okay. Relax and set a new goal for the next day. You are not here to shame yourself for being unable to do normal activities. But you want to do your best to focus on your well-being. Movement is so good for mental health and for detoxification. The more you can move those toxins out of your body, the better you will feel! Just do your best!

6. **Get into your meditation practice!**
Practice gratitude and fill yourself with love. Use guided imagery to move the cancer out of your body. See Chapter 9 for examples. I imagined my cancer being filled with love until it disintegrated. I would also pretend that I shot lasers at them until they disappeared. YouTube is an amazing source for guided imagery to heal cancer. Choose one that resonates with you!

Also, meditation can help you relax and become present. I found it helpful for relieving stress and calming the scary internal chatter.

7. **Make a list of questions for your oncologist.**
We don't always know what questions to ask our oncologist. Chris Wark is a colon cancer survivor who used holistic therapies to beat his cancer. His list of questions is useful for your first visit to an oncologist. Remember that this is YOUR choice if you choose to do conventional treatments. If you choose to support yourself through holistic therapies, make sure your oncologist is on board. https://www.chrisbeatcancer.com/wp-content/uploads/2015/12/20-Questions-For-Your-Oncologist.pdf

Make sure that you have a complete understanding of the worst possible side effects you may experience, and get a list of all of the over-the-counter medications that can offer you support.

8. **Ask to speak with a social worker at your cancer center for resources** on financial assistance, information on power of attorney and wills and support groups. They may even provide exercise classes, mental health support, nutrition services and other complimentary services. Check in with your nurse navigator and/or social worker at your cancer center. Utilize as many resources as possible!

9. **Questions for surgeon.**
   Having breast surgery can be a very emotional decision. It is important to understand your surgery options and what is best for your cancer staging. Ask about the risk of recurrence when weighing out your options. Weigh your options and possible out-of-pocket expenses for breast reconstruction, should you have a mastectomy. Each case is different. Some patients have surgery first, some have to go through chemo-therapy. Make sure your surgeon explains their decision as to why your surgery is performed before or after chemotherapy. If you would rather not do chemotherapy, ask what the risks are to opt for surgery only instead of chemo-therapy. There are many different ways this can

be done, but this also can depend on how far your cancer has progressed.

Make sure you have an understanding of how much time your surgery requires for healing so that you can assemble a team of people to offer help during that time.

Find out any possible side effects and pains you may experience so that you can combat them with the right supplementation and/or over-the-counter medications.

10. **Assemble your holistic team.**

It can be very expensive to work with a naturopath; this is why I mention getting books to support you in this journey. I also recommend finding support groups through Facebook that focus on integrative care. Many of these groups have a wealth of data and information on supplementation and bloodwork that you might be able to get your oncologist to do. Some oncologists are open to providing certain blood tests; however, not all understand why. Remember, they are not trained in holistic health. They are tumor experts and Doctors of Medicine. This is not a part of their education. This is why I do suggest working with a naturopath as they are aware of testing that can keep you healthy through your treatments and assist you should you decide not to do conventional treatments.

Acupuncture is very supportive through cancer and can be done rather inexpensively if you can find a place that does community acupuncture. Note that if you do community acupuncture, you may want to find out when they experience slow times and go then. Remember that when you receive conventional treatments, your blood counts drop, leaving you at risk for getting sick easily. Take extra precautions when going. Sanitize your hands before and after your arrival. You can also wear a mask for safety.

II. **Meeting with a radiation oncologist.**
How anyone reacts to radiation varies from person to person. Your skin can possibly suffer burns and you may experience tightness in the underlying tissues. It can feel sore and lumpy where radiated. Also, if you have lymph nodes that were removed and radiation to those areas, you'll want to find out if there are lymphedema specialists at your cancer center that can help you understand what lymphedema feels like and how to treat it. Make sure that your radiation oncologist prescribes you a cream to apply after your radiation appointments and throughout the day. Gather as much information as possible on how to treat burns. Ask about how to proceed with exercise, especially

in the case where you may be at risk for lymph-edema. Ask for the worst-case scenario on side effects. Having a better understanding of how you might respond to treatment allows you to plan ahead for meal deliveries and other assistance you may need during that time. Many people experience fatigue. Allow yourself the time and space to take naps.

12. **How to feel beautiful when bald!**
What makes you feel beautiful? Is it wearing bold clothing? I have a coat that my partner calls the celebrity coat. When I wear it, everyone stops to look at it. Some run up and want to touch it or ask where I bought it. It is a delightful conversation piece.

You can empower yourself through this journey when you feel like your beauty is fading away.

Wear clothing that makes you feel good! I wore sundresses and sandals with cute hats and big, bold earrings and wound beautiful scarves around my head. Wear something that you feel powerful in. Your hair doesn't make you, your spirit does! Shine your light bright and be bold! Throw on some sparkles and bedazzle yourself!

Your skin can get super dry during chemo-therapy. Drink lots of water and keep your skin moisturized at all times. Sometimes oil-based cleansers and serums are best during chemo. My skin store has amazing products for dehydration. www.studioskinandtonic.com

Find your favorite bright lipsticks!

Get some vibrant wigs or something that feels right for you! I barely wore wigs because they were too itchy BUT I loved scarves and caps. There are many places you can get them. Your cancer center may have resources to get them at discounted costs. This website has amazing caps, hats and other beauty support for your journey. https://www.headcovers.com/gifts-catalog/cancer-gifts/

Magnetic lashes are another wonderful way to keep your feminine looks intact! There are many places you can choose from. I used Glamnetics and was very pleased! https://www.headcovers.com/gifts-catalog/cancer-gifts/

Brow tattoos preserved my sanity. My penciled brows always ended up lopsided. I purchased sheets of brow tattoos from Insta Eyebrows https://www.instaeyebrows.com/

You can line them up perfectly on your face, place a hot compress over the top for one minute and remove. Voilà, you have brows for a few days! The brows will last longer per use if you can avoid scrubbing that area of your face!

Because I'm a weirdo, I would draw crazy brows on my face and do characters. I dressed up as Charlie Brown for Halloween. I needed to have some humor around it and make myself laugh. Dress up as Mr. Clean! I dressed up as a fortune teller and gave video palm readings during the pandemic! Lean into it and be ridiculous! Remember that this is only temporary!

13. **Have an open conversation with your partner about EVERYTHING.**

Your body is going to experience a lot of things that feel awful. Losing your hair and dry skin is part of it. Your libido may disappear. I forgot about sex during my cancer treatment and even after. Before cancer I was always ready for sex even when I wasn't ready. Chemotherapy kicked me right into menopause, which did not help. I stopped thinking about sex. I discovered vaginal atrophy. Vaginal atrophy is thinning and inflammation of the vaginal walls and can make sex very painful. Water-based lubricants caused a lot of stinging and discomfort. I found that oil or oil-based suppositories and lubricants really helped. Woo Organic Coconut Oil is great for softening and lubricating the vaginal walls. I recommend a towel underneath, so you don't get oil everywhere! https://woomoreplay. com/products/coconut-love-oil

Have an open conversation about sex with your partner. You can find ways to have intimacy and fun without having sex. My partner and I scheduled what we called naked days. We enjoyed exploring and finding new ways to be intimate. I found that it brought us closer too! We had conversations that allowed us to both feel heard about our needs and together found solutions that kept us both happy.

Check in with each other regularly around everything happening in your cancer journey. Your partner is going through their own thoughts and emotions and under constant worry. You can find ways to support each other that can really bring you together. Therapy and support groups can also be helpful. Your cancer center may have programs to support you and your partner as you go through your journey.

I truly hope that you find this book helpful. I wish you all the love, health, and healing in your journey!

Afterword

I swear I was going to be done doing the cancer thing this year, but apparently, there was more. All things considered, I have come out of this whole debacle on top and alive.

I've always said I'm one of those type A, LET'S DO ALL THE THINGS AND MAKE SHIT HAPPEN, but I wasn't talking about sampling the cancer smorgasbord. I mean REALLY?

At the end of February, I was still having a rough recovery after the last round of radiation. I wasn't healing and I was in a lot of pain but oddly a lot of head pain. LOTS of pain plus vertigo. I couldn't drive, couldn't walk and had constant spins. I did not sign up for being drunk 24/7!

Just 2 months out of radiation, My PET scan indicated everything was clear. PET scans use glucose for helping detect cancer. Cancer feeds off glucose and lights up the areas on the body where the cancer begins to absorb that fuel. Here's the thing!!! The brain uses a lot of glucose on its own so sometimes these scans are less than super accurate for detecting brain tumors.

The week after I had my PET scan, admitted myself to the ER to find out why the walls were spinning and why the pain in my head and neck was so terrible. CT scan and MRI confirmed a little mass in my cerebellum. Lucky for me, not life-threatening, plus, bonus, the very best place for a tumor since it doesn't effect cognitive function, among other really important brain functions like eating, seeing, hearing and so on. My problem was severe vertigo and feeling like utter shit. Which was the good news.

After several hours in the East Bay ER, I was transported to UCSF to work with one of the best neurosurgeons on staff. After days in the hospital, I had brain surgery. VOILA! That sucker was removed without much trouble. Not bad for brain surgery!

I'm going to live! Yes! Live like I always live, whole heartedly without a doubt, toting around my yodeling pickle and astonishing passersby. It's my life's purpose!

After this run, I'm done doing cancer and decided to get a different hobby!!! Maybe shelf painting, stamp collecting, pickle pipping. Ha!

But really, I'm going to continue writing because I've been on the path to miraculous, awesome healing and it is my destiny to show my audience the many ways to rock your life through any illness. All you need are the right tools.

I hope that you'll be waiting on the other side, mouths watering, wondering what this tiny human with a big zest for life has in store for you. Just know, there are never any dead ends and the pathways to wellness and healing while twisty, can have a totally happy destination. I'VE GOT YOU!!!

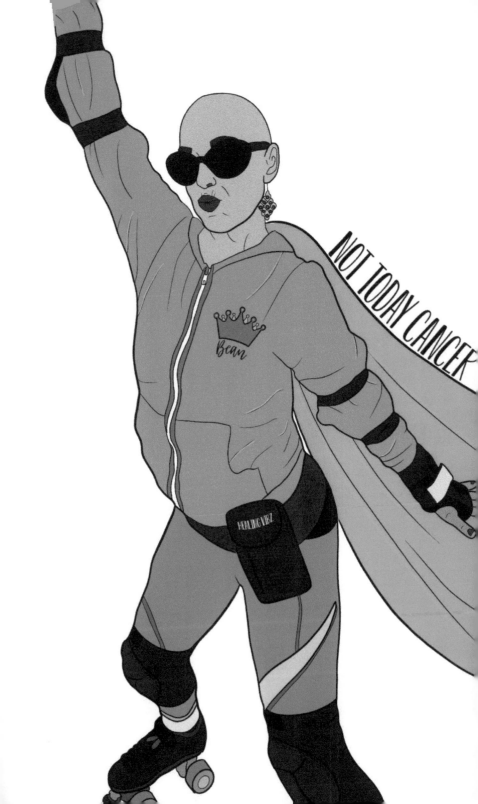